Fit 2 Love

"*Fit 2 Love* is not your typical weight ⸺ o finding authentic love that starts with your re ⸺ body."

⸺ .D., author,
Power Over Food

"A fun, inspiring and practical guide on fitness and love. *Fit 2 Love* is sure to help you attract love, while you create a deeper relationship with your body."

– Relationship expert MARYANNE COMAROTO,
Founder of the National Action Organization
"Changing the way our culture values women."

"JJ Flizanes is a leader in the fitness industry and she uses science as her background. I trust her depth of knowledge and matter of fact attitude. *Fit 2 Love* will change your body and your relationships."

– JONNY BOWDEN, PhD, CNS,
board-certified nutritionist and best-selling author,
The 150 Healthiest Foods on Earth and *The Most Effective Ways to Live Longer*

"*Fit 2 Love* is an engaging, uplifting, easy to follow guide to creating the life and body you love and then shows you how to attract the love of your life, too. Filled with great stories and illuminating tips and strategies, you will be motivated and inspired to love yourself while you improve yourself!

– CHELLIE CAMPBELL, author,
"The Wealthy Spirit" and *"Zero to Zillionaire"*

JJ is a passionate advocate for not only fixing your body but healing the inside and the outside and more importantly she lives her own truth - a rare commodity in the "diet" industry. She is thoughtful, intelligent, and considers all possibilities when guiding people in their own journey back to fitness, health, and wellness. *Fit 2 Love* is a book you must read!

– AJAY ROCHESTER
Author of Confessions of a Reformed Dieter and
The Lazy Girl's Guide to Losing Weight and Getting Fit.
Celebrity Blogger for Diet.com
- Ajay Rochester has Been There Done Fat™

"How we feel about our bodies has everything to do with how we feel about ourselves and our lovability. *Fit 2 Love* is a must read for any woman who wants to experience more love in her life. Your friends will tell you to love yourself more, but *Fit 2 Love* will make it happen!"

– MORGANA RAE
Author of *Financial Alchemy: Twelve Months of Magic and Manifestation*

"JJ Flizanes is passionate about the power of fitness and self care to transform your health and your love life. She is living proof that her formula works. If you are ready for a transformation, then, Fi*t 2 Love*, is your prescription!"

– ALLEN PETERS
M.D. of Nourishing Wellness Medical Center

"*Fit 2 Love* is the most important concept for single or unhappy married women everywhere. JJ's 5 steps can improve anyone's life and relationships- I love this book!"

– ADOLEY ODUNTON, author,
*Confessions of an Adrenaline Addict:
How to Achieve More with Less Effort*

"In her new book, *Fit 2 Love*, JJ presents a new perspective to the way we workout: body mind, and spirit. She has come up with five steps to transform both your body and your love life. Start now!"

– LISSA COFFEY, *author,
CLOSURE,
the Law of Relationship*

"A practical guide on fitness and love that is fun and inspiring. *Fit 2 Love* can help you attract love, while you create a deeper relationship with your body."

– CONNIE UMBENHOWER, *author,
The Deity Diet,
founder of Himalayan Bootcamp*

"Whether you are looking for love or just want to have a better relationship with your body, JJ's 5 steps in *Fit 2 Love* will definitely transform your body and your life. JJ's passion and plea for the best life you can live is heartfelt on every page."

– JEANNE PETERS
RD of Nourishing Wellness Medical Center

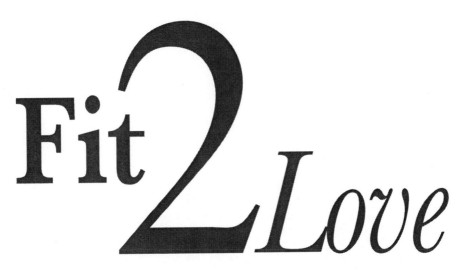

Fit 2 Love

How to get physically, emotionally, and
spiritually fit to attract the love of your life

JJ Flizanes

Fit 2 Love
JJ Flizanes

Copyright© 2010
All rights reserved.
ISBN: 978-0-9827465-6-1
Library of Congress Control Number: 2010942854

Printed in the United States of America
Bush Street Press
237 Kearny Street, #174
San Francisco, CA 94108
www.bushstreetpress.com
press@bushstreetpress.com

Cover Design by Greg Albers

The information provided in this book is designed to provide helpful information on the subjects discussed. This book is not meant to be used, nor should it be used, to diagnose or treat any medical condition. For diagnosis or treatment of any medical problem, consult your own physician. The publisher and author are not responsible for any specific health or allergy needs that may require medical supervision and are not liable for any damages or negative consequences from any treatment, action, application or preparation, to any person reading or following the information in this book. References are provided for informational purposes only and do not constitute endorsement of any websites or other sources. Readers should be aware that the websites listed in this book may change.

I dedicate this book to Gus and Valerie Flizanes, my parents, for embodying the examples of love, respect, kindness, and humility. You set the bar for what to expect and desire in a marriage, and I am grateful to have been raised by both of you. You are amazing people, wonderful parents, and a gift to this world. I love you very much and thank you from the bottom of my heart.

I also dedicate this book to my husband, Brian Albers, for being the one I was waiting for all my life. Without you, I could not have written this book. Thank you for your collaboration with this project, your love and affection, and for just being you—who is perfect for me. I will be forever grateful for all your love and support. I love you, H!

Acknowledgments

Many people made this book possible to bring to print at this particular time in my life. I am grateful to have so many people to turn to and say thank you. Alan Greenstadt, I thank you for your belief in the project. I would not have come this far without your support.

To Phil Alberstat, for your undying support and the idea that sparked this new brand; Alicia Dunams, my publisher, for your hard work, diligence, guidance and patience with me.

Greg Albers, my graphic designer, for your craftsmanship of the inside and outside. Thank you for your willingness and patience to work around my crazy deadlines.

Rudi Parcon, my photographer, for an amazing photo shoot and scenic tour of Miami. Thank you for all you did to help get this done. Edwin Verdezoto, from Royal Flowers, for the gorgeous roses that appeared in all my shots. The roses also made my stay in Miami while finishing this book extra beautiful!

Tracy Coe, from Body Mind Coe-Dynamics Pilates Studio, for all your Pilates help for this book. I look forward to working together on more projects.

Carol Chanel, my coach, for your amazing insight and coaching through all my relationships over the last several years. You were the first person to call and celebrate when Brian and I found each other. I love you and thank you for always being there.

Macarena Bianchi, I thank you a million times over for your poem, your editing, your referrals to make this project happen, and everything else in between. You are much more than my editor, of course, you are one of my best friends. I love you!

Brian Albers, Alexis Neely, Jody Lay, Jennifer and Aaron Torok, Mike Burrichter and Casey Capshaw, for your willingness to share your stories and in some cases, bare your souls. It's through your stories that others can get a taste of what is possible and find hope if they have lost it. Thank you for your participation in this movement.

Bibi Goldstein, Cathy Alessandra, Kelly Abajano, Susan Grady, Janice Gallardo, Jennifer Kwon, Jenny Buckles, Midge Ebben, Valerie Flizanes and Brian Albers, for being my support team at every stage.

Brian Albers, my loving husband, for your patience, participation, and overall support of me, us, this and our life together. I could not do any of this without you.

Contents

Introduction

"Do you want to meet the love of your life? Look in the mirror." **Byron Katie**

It's a beautiful, warm, sunny day in Los Angeles, and I have just arrived at a local gym to train one of my clients. It's business as usual as I walk in the door and head to the stretching area to meet my appointment, until I stop dead in my tracks and look around the room; I notice a strange energy in the air.

Today seems different.

As I look around the midsize gym, I see a few famous actors who are wearing their sunglasses while they workout. Celebrity sightings are common, and the locals know to leave them alone, but today, for some strange reason, I can't stop staring at them.

Are they afraid that people will come up to them? Do they not realize that we know who they are and that they call more attention to themselves by wearing sunglasses in the gym? Or maybe, they secretly want to be noticed so they try to look cool, yet uninterested.

If they want attention, they are not alone.

Heavy breathing across the room from the trainers who are power lifting catches my attention. Intense physical work needs a greater amount of oxygen than a normal workout and maybe even some sound, but I am not the only one noticing that they are putting on a show. Heavy weights being thrown on the floor, lots of shouting and almost screaming fills the corner of the gym where the dumbbell rack resides.

As I look toward the machine circuit, I see a few female trainers wearing next to nothing. *How does baring it all correlate to their knowledge and skill as a trainer?* They look around the room to see who is checking them out, while my concern is for their client with the heavy weights in their hands. The female trainers seem more interested in the attention than being present and attentive.

The vibe in the air is so thick and uncomfortable; I can almost smell and taste it. What is it? Ah, yes, it is insecurity. You could step into almost any gym and witness this scene for yourself on any given day, but today is the day I can't ignore it any longer. I can actually feel many people working out as if their life depended upon it. I can hear them saying to themselves, *I have to look perfect or no one will love me. I have to look perfect or no one will hire me.* I can sense competition, comparing, judgment, and fear. This is probably why I have not been training in gyms for a long time because the vibe makes me sad.

There are three things in life that people spend a great deal of time, money, and effort to achieve: love, health, and money. Are you single and looking for love? Do you desire a better relationship from your partner and even yourself? Do you struggle with weight loss and body issues? If you have said *yes* to just one of these questions, then you will be delighted because this book was created to help you achieve love and security through fitness and health.

The Love of Your Life is You

To love yourself means believing in your own worthiness, as well as caring for every facet of your life. Without loving yourself first, you set up a rollercoaster of dependency upon other people to make you feel good. Just like with any substance addiction, the search for love to fulfill us can spiral out of control and cause unnecessary heartache. There is another way.

There is no other set of words as perfect about self-love than the poem

Our Deepest Fear, which inspires me to tears every time I read it. It's by Marianne Williamson from *A Return To Love: Reflections on the Principles of A Course in Miracles*:

> Our deepest fear is not that we are inadequate. Our deepest fear is that we are powerful beyond measure... Your playing small does not serve the world. There is nothing enlightened about shrinking so that other people won't feel insecure around you. We are all meant to shine,...

How I Got Here

I have been in the fitness industry for close to 15 years and started out the way every trainer is supposed to, by taking classes and getting certified. For most trainers, that's all there is to it. I always want to go deeper, learn more, and discover the infamous *truth* behind it all.

Before becoming a trainer, I was a performer. As a singer, dancer, and actor, I studied human behavior and motivation through relationships created on stage and screen. I was interested in the study of people, which is why I studied acting. I learned more about myself and my own psychology, religion, politics, and history through one of my acting classes at NYU in 1992 than I did in traditional school. It was an amazing experience to be able to look through someone else's eyes, the character, and see life from a different perspective. It gave me such insight and helped me to look inside myself in a different way. I was hooked.

The study of people and how they work has always intrigued me, so it was a natural transition to use my acting background and apply it to help people change their body and lives through personal training. I had no idea when I started studying exercise science that I would love the science of the body so much. I went from thinking I was only a creative person who was not good at science and math to loving the application of science on the body because I could see it! Then I began to teach it. I ran the education department of a major gym chain on the East Coast for almost two years, using my performing background to inspire other trainers to greater knowledge of the body so we could all help our clients get the body they wanted in a safer, more effective way.

In the last two decades, I have studied biomechanics, anatomy, physiology, biochemistry, personalities, psychology, human interaction and behavior, astrology, and spirituality. Every year, I learned a little bit more, I dug a little bit deeper, and asked different questions about the sciences I was learning, none of which answer the very basic, *brass taxes*, bottom-line question: what was really the most motivating factor in achieving success with the body? The biggest key ingredient in having success with your body, fitness, happiness, and life boils down to one thing: self-love.

Now, you may think that may be oversimplifying it, but I invite you to open up to the possibility that it may be true. There have been 15 years of research on human behavior and the different applications of my work and their results. I can use my own life as an example through my transformation from a little girl to an independent woman, including how I treated myself and my own evolution of finding my own love, my perfect mate, my knight in shining armor and the steps that I had to go through to get here—and get him!

Looking at my life, including my blueprints, experiences, and processes, it is clear that the steps I took that changed my life can be applied to everyone. They will work for you, whether you are looking for a mate or need to love yourself more completely.

While there is no one way to find your ideal mate, what's been noticeable over and over in friends, clients, and myself is that quality relationships start from a place of respect and independence. Each person needs a degree of self-respect and has to have a solid and happy life independent from their partner.

I am going to help you create a blueprint and strategy of how you can manifest your perfect mate—the one you long to be with forever. You will learn how to use the everyday actions that maintain your body, like eating and exercising, to bring you more love, whether it be from another person or from yourself.

A lifetime of experience has taught me what works and what doesn't work. I've lived it. At the end of the day, all we want to do is be happy and feel the love that we know is possible. I look forward to sharing this experience with you and hearing about the success that you attain along the way.

Chapter 1

Your Body Blueprint

"Your relationship with yourself is the central template from which all others are formed. Loving yourself is a prerequisite to creating a successful and authentic union with another."
Dr. Cherie Carter-Scott

One of the tools that was pivotal in helping me manifest and manage all my relationships since 1998 was Dr. Cherie Carter-Scott's book, *If Love is a Game, These are the Rules.* It was the first time I really understood the concept that how others treated me was a direct result of how I treated myself. When I could stand back and be objective about my behavior toward myself and what messages that sent out to others, I realized that the relationship I had to focus on most to get what I wanted was with myself. If I was not willing to treat myself like a queen, then how could I expect someone else to?

Your turn.

How do you treat yourself? When you wake up in the morning, what do you say to yourself? Do you compliment or criticize your body? Do you try on clothes, pinpointing all of the negative things you can, secretly wishing you could have someone else's body?

If you do, you are not alone. This common practice of most women is the exact behavior that drives the fitness and weight loss industry—and I hate it. We focus on perfect bodies and *how can I spot reduce this area so I will like myself, or so someone else will find me attractive and valuable?* The underlying emotion here is fear. Many spiritual teachers of mine over the years have all agreed that our actions are motivated consciously or subconsciously by either love or fear.

Fear is defined as *a feeling of agitation and anxiety caused by present or imminent danger and a feeling of disquiet or apprehension.* Fear can be a good tool when you think your life is in danger, but most people live in this emotion all day long with no such threat. Fear is uncomfortable to be in and around. Fear can also be defined as lack of trust.

Love is defined as *a deep, tender feeling of affection and care toward a person, such as that arising from kinship or a sense of oneness, and a person who is the object of deep or intense affection or attraction.* Love feels good, and we seek it all the time. We hold others as objects of our attention to give love to, and we want to receive love from others.

Which of these is activated more in your life when you deal with your body? Is it mostly love or fear?

How many times in your relationship life do you attract people who do the same thing or change the way they treat you as the relationship progresses? They start off complimentary and wonderful in the first two or three months, then the compliments stop coming because you either did not receive them or you argued about them.

You trained them how to treat you.

How often do you deflect a compliment? Someone tells you that you look pretty, and you say, "Oh no, I just rolled out of bed, and I am having a bad hair day." This blocks a compliment.

Many women do it because they have a hard time receiving. You are not allowing yourself to receive the gift because your inner critic does not believe what the other person says. You *want* to feel attractive, then someone gives you a compliment, and you reject it. Can you see what message you are sending to that person? Why would anyone compliment you again?

Take out a sheet of paper and answer these questions to see what your body blueprint says about you based on every area of fitness and self-care, including exercise, diet, rest, play, and self-talk. We will then work on creating a new body blueprint that can yield more desirable responses.

1. List all the thoughts you can remember you had today, from the time you woke up to now, about how you look or any judgments on your character. For example, if you made a mistake, did you quickly internalize with a thought like *"I am so stupid,"* or did you think *"Oh well, glad I learned that now?"* List all of your thoughts in a single column.

2. Underneath the last thought, write a list all the actions you did today, from taking a shower to eating breakfast. Also include things you would have like to have done or should have done and didn't. For example, you did not take your supplements today.

You should have one long vertical row that contains all the thoughts you were aware of today and all the actions you have accomplished so far. Now make another column to the right of the first one and answer these questions.

1. Next to the thoughts you had, write down if they were positive comments or negative. If you criticized yourself, that is negative. If you brushed your teeth, that is positive.

2. Next to the actions, write down a brief reason for doing that action and whether it came from love or fear. For example, if you wrote down 'had a cup of coffee, went to work and skipped breakfast,' do you think skipping breakfast was an act of love or disregard? You know the body needs fuel, so if the reason you skipped breakfast was because you were too busy, you put work before yourself, which sends the message that you are not as important as your work. Keep going through your list and be honest with yourself about the messages you are sending.

What Does Your Body Blueprint Say?

Answer the questions below and identify the message you are sending with each of your answers.

1. Exercise: How do you take care of your body? Do you exercise regularly? What kind of exercises do you do and why?

2. Diet: What foods do you consume on a regular basis? Are they high energy, clean foods that provide vitamins and nutrients for your body? Are they processed, chemically created foods that contain large amounts of fat and sugar with no nutritional value? Do you consume the amount of water your body needs to function optimally every day? Do you ingest toxins and drugs?

3. Rest: Do you sleep at least seven to eight hours a day? Do you unwind before going to bed? Do you take breaks during the day to relax and recharge your mind and body?

4. Play: Do you have fun on a weekly basis? Do you laugh often? Do you feel joy and do things you love every week?

5. Self-talk: How do you treat yourself with the words you use in your mind? If you talked to someone else the way you talk to yourself, how would they respond?

The thoughts you are aware of and your actions are part of your consciousness. You can change those behaviors starting now. But before we start to focus on the steps of changing your body blueprint to build the kind of relationships you want in your life, let's acknowledge how some of these habits got there in the first place. Why is it this way? Where did these patterns of thought come from?

Your Subconscious Mind

Your subconscious mind was formulated from the time you were born up until about eight years old. Often referred to as the basement of your mind, those beliefs were put there whether you were aware of it or not. They have been stored in the basement of your mind your entire life and drive all the thoughts and feelings that you have now—this is the subconscious mind. The subconscious mind makes up 88% of your thoughts and beliefs, whereas the conscious mind is only 12%. As you can deduce, the subconscious mind is running your life. I collaborated on a course called the *6 Week Body Program*, where we help you reprogram your subconscious mind easily and effortlessly through the use of creative visualization and hypnosis. It's easy, painless, and starts to clean out that basement in your mind. Working with hypnosis in general can help uncover subconscious beliefs and patterns and help you to easily replace any old negative beliefs with new and more supportive ones. When wanting to deal with your subconscious, you will need assistance of some kind.

Attending to your conscious mind is something you can start doing immediately. I would not recommend trying to adjust everything on the list at the same time. Pick one of the five areas listed above and number them in the order that would be the best place for you to start.

Changing Your Body Blueprint

Here are some suggestions of tools you can use for each of the self care categories.

1. Exercise: Get a buddy. Schedule exercise into your week. Hire a fitness coach or personal trainer. Join a gym. Start an exercise group in your area to hold yourself accountable while socializing with some friends and neighbors. Take some time to find out why you don't exercise and find something you *will* do that might look like exercise. You can exercise in many different ways, and a gym is not necessary. Keep a self-care journal and write down the physical activity you do each day.

2. Diet: Clean out your refrigerator and pantry. Buy a healthy cookbook. Schedule and plan your meals. Hire a chef. Swap fast food for healthy alternatives at the grocery store. Pack your

lunch and snacks. Keep a food log to see what you are choosing to eat. Do a detoxification. Find a local farmer's market. Order home-delivered fresh produce from a farm. Spend the money on home-delivered fresh meals daily to help with portion control, calories, and nutrients. Plan to eliminate one toxic thing from your diet each week. Carry healthy snacks so you can always maintain your blood sugar and energy. Try a new vegetable every week. Eat protein at every meal.

3. **Rest:** Sleep at least seven hours every night, and create a ritual to transition from living your day to resting your body. Take a bath before bed. Drink some herbal tea. Write in a journal and offload any lingering ideas or thoughts to clear your mind. Use a self massager to relax your muscles and wind your body down. Turn off all electronics and be still in the quiet for few minutes before falling asleep. Use your mind to relax every part of your body from your feet to your head. Listen to hypnosis while you wind down to help change the subconscious mind and relax your body into sleep.

4. **Play:** Schedule a play date at least two or three times a week with family or friends. Pick things you want to do that get you excited, just like when you were a child. Make a list of all the fun things you would love to do without reasoning money or time. Research events in your area that might be free or low cost. Create a savings account or piggy bank for your adventures or travel. Pin up a map on the wall and mark all the places you want to go or make a list of things you want to see. Create a play vision board with pictures from magazines, and then number them in the order you want to accomplish them. Make a plan to do each one. Laugh every day.

5. **Self-talk:** Use a daily journal to make a list of positive aspects about yourself every day. List your accomplishments, as well as positive character traits you displayed each day. Use affirmations. Ask your friends and family what they love about you and read one response to yourself every day. Get a therapist or coach. Use hypnosis or the *6 Week Beach Body Program*.

You will see the transformation of many of the people I spoke with about *Fit 2 Love*. When they changed their body blueprint, they attracted the love into their life that they had always wanted. Some of that love came from another, but the love that mattered most was the one that came first from themselves.

Over the course of my life thus far, I have had to learn how to quiet my inner critic, replace those thoughts with more supportive and loving behavior, and practice putting myself first as often as possible. With or without a partner, you are the only person who has to live with yourself for the rest of your life. My desire was to be as happy as I could with me, myself, and I. When I got there, I attracted my perfect mate because I had already found the love of my life within myself.

Chapter 2

Manifesting My Husband in 3 Weeks

"Plant your own garden and decorate your own soul, instead of waiting for someone to bring you flowers." Veronica A. Shoffstall

My dating history is pretty standard, with many short relationships and a few long-term relationships, which lasted from one to four years. I was a "one man" kind of woman for most of my life. Each time the relationship came to an end, I trusted that I was supposed to learn something from it about myself or change in some way to better prepare for *the one.*

You have two options when a relationship ends. The negative, self-destructive option would be to feel helpless, victimized, and as if the world is going to end. *Why did this happen to me? What am I going to do now?*

This option is easier in many ways because it puts blame on someone or something else, and that is highly acceptable in our culture. You can conveniently make it *not about you* to avoid looking in the mirror and owning where you are and what you have attracted into your life. The problem becomes when you keep attracting the same kind of relationship over and over again and keep thinking it's always the other person's fault.

The road less traveled is to practice having trust in a bigger plan and divine timing. Each relationship serves you in some way; you attract it based on where you are. Learn from it, grow more into who you really are, and then move on.

The only thing you are in control of is *you*.

You get to decide how to look at things, how you react, and what you do about it. It's not always easy to look inside and question. It takes love and trust.

Being the analyst that I am, I would often want to identify my lessons from the relationship as soon as possible after it ended. This way, I could justify my invested years with each partner in order to feel a sense of accomplishment, instead of failure. I wanted to be able to appreciate the time I spent, the lesson learned, and have no negative energy around it so I could move on with love and gratitude.

Failure is not an option in my world; evolution is. Sometimes you have to breakdown in order to breakthrough.

On February 5, 2006, I met my husband. The background story is that I was already in a relationship, as well as secretly still in love with my ex-boyfriend. My plate was full, and I was not actively looking for another man. As the old adage says, it happens when you least expect it.

It was a bright, sunny Sunday afternoon at a party in Tustin, California, where the guest list consisted of mostly Pittsburgh Steelers Fans gathering to watch the Super Bowl. The hosts were former clients of mine that I had not seen in many months. I was looking forward to visiting with them. Once settled in at the party, I engaged in girl talk until the door opened downstairs and this wave of energy walked into the room.

I sensed it before I saw him—it was very strange and the first time I had ever experienced something like that.

Taken by this energy, I turned around to see who it was, and there was this handsome, clean cut, yet slightly edgy guy carrying some snacks up the stairs.

The first thing I noticed is that he was attractive.

He was carrying a bag of chips in one hand and a Pyrex dish in the other. The tightly and almost perfectly Saran-wrapped Pyrex dish had salsa inside with six perfectly-cubed pieces of Velveeta cheese evenly spaced in three rows of two.

This guy is organized and precise.

He was wearing khaki's, a button-down shirt, and a baseball cap—very jock-like, until I noticed the silver jewelry. He had one silver ring on each hand and a silver bracelet around his right wrist.

This guy is sensitive.

Men that wear jewelry are often more comfortable with their sexuality and are in touch with their feminine side. They also tend to be romantic and sensitive.

I was assessing every move. *Very interesting, seems like a punk. He's cute, but I'd never date him.* It was an interesting experience to notice him and decide that nothing could come of it because of my various reasons.

The party went on. I visited with my friends and was only paying half attention to the game since I don't follow any particular team. I was born into being a Steelers Fan, and that got me a ticket to the party. I was most interested in socializing.

He was not paying attention to me at all; he was watching the game. I was growing more curious about him, so I pulled out the laptop and asked if I could do his astrological chart. (It was the sneaky way to find out more about him and see if there was interest in exchanging email addresses). He agreed, and away I went with my astrological inspection. Excited to find out he was a Pisces like me, I rattled off the details of my findings. He was interested but still focused on the game, so I offered to email it to him. Nothing else really happened that night because I had made plans after the party with the other men in my life (they were both at the same function), so I left earlier than everyone else.

After the weekend, I wondered about him. Now you must know that I have a detailed list of what *I want* and *do not want* in a partner that I have been editing and revising since 1998. My list was a tool I learned from Dr Cherie Carter-Scott's book, *If Love is A Game, These are the Rules*. I was on my sixth or seventh edition of this list since its creation, and Brian had two things that fell in the "deal breaker" category, so in my conscious, intellectual mind, this match would never materialize. Yet, something made me wonder.

I called my friends and asked, "Did he ask about me?"

To which they replied, "No."

"Well, I need you to have another party so I can see if there is something here between us, okay?"

And so, they did. Two weeks later, we had the "come finish our beer" party, which was a slightly smaller group without the focus on the TV, so now his attention could be on me. We sat at a table together, where he proceeded to try and teach me a card game while we consumed a bottle of red wine, ate pizza and chocolate covered sesame seeds, and conversed about astrology. I could tell he was into me. The party went on around us as sparks were flying, and we got lost in our own world of philosophy, astrology, and red wine.

Over the weekend, I came to find out that he called our friends this time and said, "Did she ask about me?"

"Yes," they replied and reported that he was extremely pleased after they confirmed my interest. This was February 17, 2006. We were both in relationships with other people, but the message was clear to me: he was interested. I know I was being clear and that he got that I was interested. The obvious next step would be to go out or get together—not quite yet.

We did not have our first date until October 28, 2006, which was approximately eight months after the time we met. *What happened?*

I am the kind of person who is normally forthcoming and aggressive. I would have had no problem calling him and asking him to do something because I knew he was interested. However, I had been studying men and relationships for ten years up to that point and learned that I wanted a real man, one who could be masculine and forthright. In order for me to get that kind of man, I needed to allow him to BE that kind of man, and not take charge. *If he is interested, he will make a move. If he does not make a move, he is either not ready or not interested.*

So, I waited.

Let me be clear, I did not wait by the phone. I was still in a relationship, still interested in my ex-boyfriend, and still curious about Brian, but I refrained from being the initiator and waited.

Well, let's not call it waiting. I lived my life.

During those eight months, the relationship I was in had ended, and I made peace with releasing my attachment to my ex-boyfriend. I did a lot of emotional work on myself to have clarity and acceptance of how I felt about the ex-boyfriend and why it didn't work, until I had new perspective and emotional response to it. Healing from heartache and broken expectations takes time and space to come to terms you can be happy about. I needed to write a new story about the next chapter in my life and start with a blank page. It was time to clean the slate and open myself up for new possibilities.

One of the ways I did this was to schedule dancing several nights a week with friends. Salsa dancing opens my heart and shuts off my brain. I need it regularly to exercise my femininity and unplug from being a business owner who operates in masculine energy most of the time. Salsa dancing is very feminine and allows me an opportunity to wear a dress, glitter, and heels! Having somewhere to go where it is encouraged (and often required) to wear frilly, sexy clothes, allowed me to express myself and have some fun.

Something I learned about relationships and myself after reading Dr Cherie Carter-Scott's book was that I was used to having companionship. One of my biggest struggles coming out of a long-term relationship was the loss of a person to hang out with on a regular basis; it really put a cramp in my social life! One of the guys I had met one night at one of my salsa clubs called me and wanted to hang out and go dancing. We became fast friends and salsa partners. We went dancing two or three times a week and often enjoyed a meal together beforehand. It was so nice to have a male companion who I could dance with and was always ready to go out when I called. It was like being in a relationship without the intimacy! I was having fun, doing what I loved, spending time with people I enjoyed, and taking care of my body; life was very good. I was happy and content.

Brian did call during the eight months, and we checked in on each other from time to time via social media and by phone. I always had him in the back of my mind, secretly hoping he would be the one. At the bottom of his MySpace page, he wrote, "Looking for the one, does anyone know where she is?" I would read that to myself when looking at his page and verbally respond aloud, "I am here. I guess you just can't see me yet."

I attended a business and personal retreat in September 2006 and used his image to create stories of the life I wanted to live and the relationship I wanted to have. I had come to terms with the fact that meeting him inspired me to dream about what was possible in a relationship and had accepted the possible reality that it might not be him. I was grateful that our conversations had given me hope and allowed me to adjust my vision about my future husband.

I created a vision board on October 3, 2006, that was centered on finding *the one*. Many people make vision boards or hang pictures of things they would like to have and think that is all you have to do; this is why it often does not work. Like exercise, you have to use the vision board every day. Using the vision board on a daily basis to practice feeling joy, love, warmth, and everything you think a relationship can give you is what make the difference in your results.

I would stand in front of my board for at least five minutes every day and focus on one picture that would get my attention and visualize myself in the picture. One of the images was a woman at a table and a man standing behind her with his arms wrapped around her and his head in her neck, as if he was going to kiss her cheek or whisper. I would study that picture, close my eyes, and FEEL the arms around me, the warm breath on my neck, and the body heat until I got a chill down my spine, as if it was really happening. Once I felt it in my body for a few minutes as if it was really happening, I would open my eyes and start my day.

After three weeks of doing this, Brian decided that it was finally time for us to meet in person once again. Our next face-to-face encounter, October 28th, lasted 28 hours. By October 31st, we had both expressed our knowing to each other that we were going to get married. We each called our parents and friends to announce that we had found the one we had been looking for all our life; this was before the second date. We were married August 9, 2008, in Princeville, Kauai.

Everyone has their own unique love story. The work I had done to set the stage for attracting this relationship can be broken down into five steps: clean the slate, sexual fitness, a food love affair, wear sexy underwear, and thank your lucky stars. If you are still writing your story, you can use the same steps that worked for me and the other men and women featured here. You will find that the biggest key to unlocking your greatest potential starts with how you take care of yourself.

Chapter 3

A Man's Point of View

"You can measure the impeccability of your word by your level of self-love. How much you love yourself and how you feel about yourself is directly proportionate to the quality and integrity of your word." Don Miguel Ruiz

Brian Albers is an architect with Jenkins, Gales, and Martinez in Los Angeles, California. He is also my husband. He was born in Green Bay, Wisconsin, and spent most of his teenage years in Toledo, Ohio. It was important to include his voice in this project because without him, my ideas are just theories and not a proven practice.

JJ: It's important for women to hear a man's perspective about his partner and his partner's blueprint. Since it was my blueprint that I worked on to attract you, it is essential to hear your point of view. I'm going to try and only call you Brian. If I slip and say *dear*, pretend you're not talking to me and that I'm somebody else asking you about your wife. Is this okay?

Brian: It's fine.

JJ: Okay, Brian, tell me a little bit about yourself, what you do for a living, something you think is interesting that people should know about you and your personality before we dive into the material.

Brian: I'm 32 years old. I'm an architect, and I'm the oldest of three boys. I have grown up having many jobs and always having to work for what I wanted to do, so I think I have a pretty strong work ethic. I was an avid athlete for most of my childhood and even still today, since I play hockey competitively, as well as participate in various outdoor activities.

JJ: When did you first start noticing you had an interest in having relationships with women?

Brian: When I was in fourth grade. I think I had my first official girlfriend in fifth grade. Her name was Kelly Van Dyke. I've always been curious and interested in the female species and being a partner in a relationship with the opposite sex.

JJ: So what was it about Kelly that struck your fancy?

Brian: She was cute: blonde hair, blue-eyed, and tall. At that age, I think I was looking for more of the exterior aesthetic package, not necessarily the romance. In fifth grade, you're not really getting romantic yet, so it was purely aesthetic from the beginning.

JJ: How long do you think you were attracted to women mostly for their looks? Men tend to be very physical and visually oriented, but at what point did something else come into the picture that was as important to consider when choosing a girlfriend?

Brian: Well, I think looks are always there. Men are visual people. Even so to this day, I'm still very attracted to you. I have a very beautiful wife, and I notice beauty all around me. Not just in women, in creatures and other living and non-living things, as well. During high school, I transformed from the physical attraction to the more emotional attraction because looks can only take you so far. When the conversation dries out or quality time is limited, there has to be a conversation. I needed to have similarities on belief systems, values, emotional integrity, and general well-being. I'm not going to want to spend a lot of time with someone that's unattractive on the inside, and you can only spend so much time with a woman that's only attractive on the outside.

JJ: Many women spend great amounts of time working on the physical aspect: trying to have the perfect body, buying the right purse, wearing the right makeup, clothes, shoes, and so on. Could you see a difference in really attractive women that didn't like themselves and tried too hard versus women that were a little bit more comfortable with themselves and maybe weren't as attractive physically?

Brian: Yes. The more attractive women were the boring ones, like the cheerleaders and party girls. The ones that I held long relationships with were the ones that in high school were not necessarily the most attractive women. It was a depth that was developed based on their personality, characteristics, and charisma that withstood the test of time better than their physical attractive qualities.

JJ: This is a passion project. It takes into account a lot of different things that I've done in my life and sort of puts them together. There are two ways to approach how we take care of ourselves: either from a place of love or a place of fear. First, we can practice self-care from a place of putting ourselves on our own pedestal of love and taking care of ourselves. The opposite motivation would be putting ourselves as the object of ridicule based on everyone else's opinions and wondering what people think to the point of letting that affect how we feel about ourselves. I'm trying to help women understand that they create the blueprint from which people treat them. Can you see any patterns of behavior toward women of your past based on how their relationship was with themselves?

Brian: For women, I think that confidence is few and far between in the early twenties. It doesn't matter whether you're attractive or the ugly duckling, I think that confidence exudes beauty. One of the reasons I was attracted to my wife was for her pure independence and confidence. I think that's a very attractive for me and for men in general. When a woman knows what she wants and who she is, that can trump the physical, because a confident woman can be as sexy, smart, and playful as she wants to be. Her inner beauty shines even brighter than her exterior qualities.

JJ: How would you describe what confidence means?

Brian: Confidence is assuredness in one's steps, whether they're forward, backwards, growing, or contracting. Confidence is assuredness in any direction.

JJ: Did you feel a definite switch from dating to *I'm ready to be a partner, I'm ready to get married?* Was there a mental switch for you?

Brian: Yes.

JJ: Before that shift happened, what did you look for in a girlfriend?

Brian: Someone to have fun with. Someone to spend quality time with and spend long hours doing things we had in common. I wanted to have fun, laugh, have adventures, and be with somebody that wanted to do the same, so I looked for common interests first and foremost.

JJ: And when you shifted, tell me about the transition from *done with girlfriends* to *now looking for a wife.*

Brian: I decided when I was 28 years old that I was sick and tired of the games. I was sick and tired of the drama and the dependency factor that girlfriends had toward me. There are all these different expectations and drama. *How is she going to act if I do this? How is he going to act to this? Why hasn't he called me? How come he's not making time for me?* I think I was just sick of all those complexities. I felt like I was responsible for bringing out the confidence in somebody else, and I didn't want that any more.

JJ: Is it safe to say that the girlfriend roles were the fun-loving, common interest, but not necessarily confident and a little bit too needy?

Brian: That's a good summary.

JJ: All right, so now you are in the transition of looking for a wife, and what are the qualities you're looking for?

Brian: I realized I didn't want to spend the rest of my life with someone that wasn't attractive inside and out. I think that there's a chemistry that develops when there's mutual attraction, which is very important to me. But above all, it was confidence. This is exactly what I said to my cat one night. I remember it very vividly because I pounded my hand so hard on the counter of my kitchen that I actually bent my ring. It's still bent today. I wanted a confident, headstrong, blonde woman from the Midwest. I think those were the four qualities that I yelled in my apartment with my cat as my witness. By headstrong, I meant confident and independent. I wanted someone from the Midwest because of the similarities and ways of growing up that I had. I've always been attracted to blondes. I don't know why. My first girlfriend was blonde, and my wife is blonde.

JJ: How did you know that you had found your wife?

Brian: I think it was a couple months after I originally met her that I realized what it was that I wanted. It was really tricky because I was actually dating someone else and growing quite bored and complacent with that person. I wanted to take that leap. I wanted to believe in a higher calling that this person was put here for me. I was going to take a jump, take a leap. I researched her on the internet and basically checked her out. I had this infatuation with this person that I'd met briefly and only spent a few hours with. I was so curious that I studied her further. I wanted to get to know her more on a personal and intimate level. I wanted to talk to her and have long phone conversations, take her out on a date, see if the signals were being received correctly. I was two months into studying her and I said, "I'm in." I called my mom and told my mom about her. I said, "I think she might be it." I had met a woman that was the perfect package: beautiful, smart, sexy, funny, and athletic. I decided that *it would work*. I knew I could be very, very happy with her.

JJ: How long after your discovery was the first date?

Brian: I had made such a profound decision in my life. I had yelled
        at my apartment walls. I got loud with my cat. I bent my ring.
        So, I took some personal time before asking her out. It was
        roughly eight months: from February to October. I wanted to
        make sure I had things prepared to make a home, create a new
        life, and start growing with her. So I took my time to clear up
        some of my past, take care of some debt, purge all of my junk
        and all of my stuff that wasn't really serving me because I was
        transitioning into a new chapter in my life. I hadn't even started
        it yet. I was so gung-ho about it that there really wasn't any
        way she was going to say no. That's how confident and sure
        of myself I was about this relationship. I knew that there was
        potential for her to be as receptive as I was. Overall, it took
        eight months. Halfway, I had made the decision. So at the four-
        month mark, I spent the rest of the rest of the time figuring out
        how to start day one.

JJ: Sounds like serious energy, attention, and planning. Many
        women on that first or second meeting are assessing the
        situation. If they don't get the follow-up call, or they don't
        get the action right away, they immediately jump to thinking
        something's wrong with them or maybe they misread the
        situation. What would you say to those women who may have
        met the right guy, but that guy's not calling? There are plenty
        of books already out there, such as *He's Just Not That Into You*,
        that encourage women to move on right away. There should be
        a level of confidence that a woman should have about her self-
        worth to not wait around.

        So here's what was going on with me during this time of eight
        months between meeting and the first date. I did not wait by
        the phone. I knew you were interested. In educating myself
        about men and the differences in masculine and feminine
        energies, I trusted that if you weren't ready, that you wouldn't
        make a move, and understood that if you weren't going to use
        the masculine energy to step up and make something happen,
        then maybe we weren't the right fit. Nevertheless, I wanted you

in my life, so I played with your image through my vision board. I wrote journal entries and created stories about us. I always just trusted that if we were meant to be, it would be.

Many women may not be at that place. The women who are searching for a husband are waiting with baited breath for the phone to ring after the first meeting or the first date if they feel sparks. They can't wait to feel more. So they behave in such ways that actually can turn men off.

I didn't know you had made a decision about me. I didn't know you knew in your mind that I was the woman you were going to marry. You gave no clues, and it was impossible to tell by your actions. What would you tell the women who have just met a guy, and they're zinging. They felt it and know that he felt it, too. Now they're dumbfounded because nothing's happening?

Brian: A love story is a very special thing between a man and a woman, which deserves patience and acceptance. It comes down to faith. It comes down to believing in a higher destiny or power that you have to search deep and hard for within yourself. Believe in the master plan, because it brings about opportunities and learning experiences.

I think it's sad to think that your life isn't complete without some other person. Had you never accepted me at the time I was ready, I would have waited. I would have waited until you were ready. In all those special love stories that you see in the movies or you read about in books, people can wait years, so eight months wasn't really a long time. Women and men nowadays are very fixated on instant gratification, and patience isn't as a strong virtue as it used to be. You need to have faith. You need to have patience and some of those classic virtues that have survived the test of time. Be patient with yourself, and be patient for what is to come.

JJ: Would you agree that the yearning comes from lack? The lack of love for one's self?

Brian: Not just lack, it is also fear. There are a multitude of reasons for a lack of confidence, faith, belief, and hope. Find the positive ways of how to be full, self-loving, self-giving, self-nurturing, and self-inviting, and all these things that bring about joy and beauty every day. When all those things are clicking and firing on all cylinders, it's like, wow, and a great sight for a man to look at! Any man will see those deeper qualities, and the good men will be more likely to fall in love with those attributes because that is something that will survive the test of time. That is a good foundation that someone can build a relationship upon. Have patience, joy, humility, and confidence.

JJ: What rules or blueprints do you think, based on knowing me, meeting me, seeing me, and studying me, do you think I put out there? How did you want to treat me?

Brian: I wanted to treat you like my queen. I wanted to care for you like the precious cherry blossom tree, something I can water and provide nutrients for your roots, till the soil around you, and help you to flourish. I can trim some of your limbs, take care of your branches, and allow your flowers to blossom. I can clean up after your leaves fall and prepare you for the next spring.

I knew that your foundation, your tree trunk, root system, and soil were very healthy. I also saw your pretty flowers and your foliage and knew I wanted to be next to that tree. I wanted to be a bird that got to sit on your limbs and just be a part of your experience.

JJ: What were some of the things that you knew would not be acceptable even before we dated?

Brian: I couldn't cut your trunk down or chop away at it; that would destroy your confidence. If I did destroy your confidence, then we would have problems. If you weren't strong enough to take the wrath of me, in my bad days, as well as my good days, that wouldn't be acceptable. I think that there's ebb and a flow between two people. It would not be fair for me to bring you down or to judge you in comparison to me. I knew that I had to fully respect you to expect that you would fully respect me in the flow of life.

JJ: How do you view women in general who take care of themselves? Can you see a difference between two attractive women, but one is confident and takes really good care of herself, while the other does not? What's the difference between those two women for you?

Brian: Yes. I can tell just by the way that they speak. You can hear the confidence in the way that a woman speaks.

JJ: I maintain the same body type, the same weight. I haven't really gone too far in either direction. If I was to go really far in one direction, let's say, I lost ten more pounds and got really lean, or I went the other way and gained weight, would that change how much you love me?

Brian: No. I can't be judgmental like that because I can also put on pounds. I have since being married. I have been going through changes personally and professionally, so I want my wife to accept me for who I am; therefore, I have to accept her for who she is as she grows and changes.

JJ: Thank you, it's important for women to hear that.

        You're an attractive and athletic male. When most women meet an attractive man, they assume that they have to look perfect. *Fit 2 Love* moves women away from thinking it has to be about what someone else thinks about them to caring more about what they think about themselves. Is it true that weight loss or weight gain will not make a big change in the way that a man sees them? What would make a big change? Is it the way a woman feels about themselves?

Brian: Oh, yeah. For example, look at Beyoncé or J-Lo. Those are thicker-bottomed women, but they work it, and everyone knows it. Men are very attracted to that. There's added poundage here or there in a woman's evolution in life, as long as she works what she's got and knows how to use it, that inner beauty comes out.

JJ: What would you tell the women searching for a quality man?

Brian: To concentrate on their foundation by building strong roots
and focusing on the things that matter. Do not be so concerned
with the trivial or minutia of life. Somebody should love you
unconditionally through all of your pregnancies, weight gain,
wrinkles, drooping, and all these different things that happen
to a woman's body. If you want unconditional love, then you
have to give yourself unconditional love first, and everything
else will fall in line. I will tell my nieces and cousins that you've
got to love yourself just the same as you want somebody else to
love you: unconditionally, truly, and deeply.

Work on the foundation, professionalism, money, work, faith,
and your hobbies. Why put pressure on yourself to find a man
in a certain time frame? Don't put any judgments or restrictions
on that. Work on yourself; be confident, sexy, and like yourself
when nobody else is looking. That's an important one to me. It
reminds me of a profound poem I heard in college called *The
Invitation* by Oriah Mountain Dreamer:

> *It doesn't interest me what you do for a living. I want
> to know what you ache for, and if you dare to dream of
> meeting your heart's longing...*

> *It doesn't interest me if the story you are telling me is
> true. I want to know if you can disappoint another to be
> true to yourself; if you can bear the accusation of betrayal
> and not betray your own soul; if you can be faithless and
> therefore trustworthy...*

And there is more. It's a very powerful poem. Find that place
and hang onto it. That's where I associate the faith, just trusting
yourself enough to know that you can make a difference. You
matter, people count on you, so you need to count on you.
That's what I would put in my foundation and will pass this on
to my nieces and my cousins.

JJ: How would you describe your wife?

Brian: From the exterior, my wife is very attractive; long, silky blonde hair, average height. I would say she is fit and tone in all the right places. She's very active. It's hard for me to keep up with her at times. She doesn't wear a lot of labels, but when she puts on these red heels that she has... Whew, she's smokin' hot!

My wife is confident. She knows *who* she is and is very strong minded as she walks about this life with a higher purpose. Sometimes, it causes her to be very forthright on what she says and what she believes. It's really a well-put-together package, and I need to thank her parents more than I do because they raised a girl who became this generous, very accepting, active, and very forgiving woman. She might be one of the kindest ladies I've ever met. She'll give you the time of day, even if she doesn't have it. She'll rescue bruised and battered animals. She gives money to the homeless. She gives and gives so much. On the inside, my wife has a lot of very unique qualities that are very special to just her. I give her an A.

JJ: Nice, I got an A. Thank you.

Brian: Well, you know, you're not shallow. I mean, she's not superficial. She doesn't need stuff. She needs to be with people. She needs the energy of having an impact on someone else's life. She strives to bring about the best in others. It's very different from me. I don't always need that human connection. I'm more of a lone wolf. I work better with inanimate objects. As long as I can do my projects, create with my hands, and build things, I'm good. She has a different kind of engine that works better with people. She is a very good daughter and a good sister. She has great relationships with her family, and her husband's family, as well, because she's a very personable person. She's very heartwarming, attentive to details, and helpful to others. She gives her quality time willingly to make somebody's life better. And, if you're lucky enough, she makes it a lot better.

JJ: Thank you, dear, for being open and willing to do this and use our experience and who we are to help better the world and help people find amazing relationships and be healthy and happy, as they're supposed to be on this planet. I love you!

Chapter 4

Step 1: Clean the Slate

"Nobody can go back and start a new beginning, but anyone can start today and make a new ending." Maria Robinson

You're tired all the time, you want to lose a few pounds quickly, and are ready for change. Enough is enough. Your body blueprint is not sending the messages you want it to, and you are ready to start over. Time to clean the slate!

We will be attending to four areas of your life to create a fresh start: your body, physical environment, emotional baggage, and current relationships.

Your Physical Body

When dealing with only the body, the first thing I recommend is a detoxification. At a physical level, proper detoxification strengthens our body's tissues and enhances the function of its systems. This can result in fast weight loss, better sleep, improved mood and focus, as well as a decrease in appetite. Detoxification is a process of removing chemicals and toxic substances from your diet, while entering into a cleansing period by eating foods that help the body eliminate built-up toxins. Not only will you be cleansing your body, you will also have the opportunity to create a new relationship with food.

Hunger is of the mind, while appetite is of the body. During a detox, you have the opportunity to become aware of the difference between hunger and appetite. Keeping a journal throughout a detox can help you become mindful at a conscious and subconscious level of how, when, what, and why you eat. With mindfulness, you get to take back control over your relationship with food.

All cleanses are not created equal, and some are not safe. While you may lose weight quickly, some encourage long durations without eating, which stresses the body, causing adrenal fatigue. Adrenal fatigue is a condition that prevents your body from recovery because your *fight or flight* response has been triggered too often for too long. Having adrenal fatigue causes weight loss resistance, which means you will have a hard time losing weight in the long run. To find out more about adrenal fatigue or to test to see if you may be affected by it, consult your local doctor that specializes in anti-aging medicine and bio-identical hormone replacement therapy.

At least three new chemicals are introduced into the planet each day, so I recommend doing a cleanse at least twice a year. In fact, we enter the world with over 200 chemicals in our body when we are born. The Environmental Working Group found that samples of blood taken from the umbilical cord of newborns contain an average of 200 chemicals that can cause cancer, brain damage, birth defects, and other serious illnesses. Our bodies have a natural detoxification system, but it is still necessary to assist our liver, colon, kidneys, and tissues at least twice a year so that our digestive system can work more effectively to eradicate these toxins from our bodies. I would recommend trying a detox on your own with the guidelines below or contacting me at 6weekbeachbody.com to find out when we host the next virtual detox group.

What to Avoid During a Detox

1. **Dairy:** Dairy is one of the top allergies that we have, and a lot of us don't even know that we're sensitive or allergic to dairy. Dairy also causes inflammation.

2. **Caffeine:** Green tea is acceptable because there's half the

amount of caffeine in green tea that there is in coffee.

3. Alcohol: Alcohol is toxic to the liver and is also a diuretic, like caffeine. It takes water out of your system. Having less water is going to make it harder for your body to perform all of its functions because your body does everything in water. It loses weight in water. It fights disease in water.

4. Gluten: Wheat is the second biggest allergy foods out of the top five. Gluten is anything made from wheat, barley, and rye. You can find it in many foods as an additive or preservative, so be sure to read labels. You can also find a list of foods containing gluten, as well as gluten-free grains in the *30 Day JUMP Start* program that you can download for free at invisiblefitness.com.

5. Fast food: Stay away from fast food, even if it's the vegetables in the fast food places. If it comes from the garden and onto your plate, that's great. If it has to sit anywhere and goes through any kind of processes and be around other chemicals, we want to stay away from it.

6. **Fried foods and packaged foods:** They have fillers and artificial preservatives that are going to make them last longer.

7. Meat: Meat can be hard on the body to digest, and we want to give your digestive system a break.

8. Salt: That doesn't mean stay away from things that have salt in them naturally, like celery. Celery can actually help lower blood pressure. Just don't add salt to your food.

9. Sugar: Sugar is another very high inflammatory agent. It's like cocaine for your body—addictive and not good for you.

10. **Artificial sweeteners, diet drinks, and diet food:** These are toxic and made with chemicals.

What to Eat During a Detox

1. **Protein:** Your protein choices are going to be fish, eggs, tofu, tempeh, edamame, or a protein powder made from peas, hemp, rice, or egg whites.

2. **Vegetables:** Have at least 3 cups everyday of different colored vegetables.

3. **Fruit:** Enjoy at least 3 servings of fruit a day.

4. **Grain:** Brown rice, white rice, quinoa, millet, amaranth, and oat.

5. **Nuts:** Almonds, walnuts, pumpkin seeds, chestnuts, cashews, and peanuts.

6. **Drinks:** Water, green tea, herbal teas that are non-caffeinated, fresh-squeezed veggie or fruit juice, and mineral water.

7. **Oils and dressings:** Vinegar, olive, grape seed, coconut, and walnut oils. Apple cider vinegar, olive oil, and a touch of mustard make a tasty homemade dressing.

8. **Snacks:** Hummus, olives, celery, carrots, dried apricots, and prunes. For example, celery with hummus or almond butter. You can mix and match anything above for a snack, as well from the protein, fruit, or veggie categories.

9. **Supplements:** Fiber, make sure to get at least 35-40 grams a day through your food or a supplement, Krill oil or Omega 3, and a probiotic.

Additional tips to help you with a detox would be to buy organic fruits and veggies locally, if possible. Make sure to sweat every day for at least ten minutes, sleep at least seven to eight hours every night, and practice stress management daily through journaling and meditation.

Your Physical Environment

When it comes to your physical environment, you should be aware of two points of view to take into consideration. The first is the organization of your space, and the second is the energy it creates, also known as Feng Shui.

Is your house neat and tidy or a mess? Can you find what you are looking for when you need it? Organization is defined as the *non-random arrangement of components or parts interconnected in a manner as to constitute a system identifiable as a unit; sequential or spatial form in which a body of knowledge, data, people, things, or other elements, is purposefully arranged.*

Having things in order, for some people, equates to feeling in control and safe. Being organized has the potential to remove underlying anxiety that may plague you from day to day. I was never the picture of perfection when it came to organization in my physical space. To be honest, I did not want to have the stress that I see most people have who are uptight about being organized. I chose to have a more relaxed outlook.

If super organized is a 10 on a scale of 1-10, and complete chaos is a 1, I have probably lived around a 5 for most of my life. I always knew where important things were and could find them under any pile, never terribly interested in cleaning just for organization sake. Since I could always find what I was looking for, why would I need to change how I kept it?

When I moved to California, I learned about Feng Shui. This is an ancient Chinese system of aesthetics believed to use the laws of both astronomy and geography to help improve one's life by receiving positive qi (pronounced "chee" and means energy). Learning how the position of my stuff could affect the energy on my body gave me a better reason to start making some changes. Space without order can cause energetic chaos that will have an effect on you emotionally and physically.

Feng Shui taught me that clutter blocks energy and flow in the area of your life that correlates with the space your clutter is in your home. Clutter had never bothered me before, until I learned it could have an effect on different areas of my life, such as relationships, money, and health.

What in your environment is creating toxins? Many of us have things that have outlived their usefulness. Are your closets and cupboards stuffed with items you don't use? Do you keep telling yourself that you will reorganize and sort through them one day soon, only one day never comes?

Clutter impacts our emotional, mental, and spiritual state. It affects not only how we feel, but also our ability to be effective. Clutter, whether it is in the form of spiritual, emotional, mental, or physical, acts like the rocks and boulders that block a river's flow and impedes the flow of our energy. Clutter drains our energy and wears down our spirit. We need energy to flow freely in order to have maximum creativity, production, expression, and satisfaction. Clutter takes away our power.

Learning about and using Feng Shui helped me to reduce my clutter and got me interested in the energy of my environment. I am still not super neat and tidy, but I still use these principles today to do the best I can. Choose which point of view works best for you and use it to clean up your physical environment.

Your Emotional Baggage

You may have negative thoughts and emotions that clog your mind and dampen your spirit. These are old ways of thinking and habits that you might not be fully aware of at this point in time. You may be holding onto emotions like resentment, anger, and guilt, which can stand in the way to your natural energy source: your body. Negative emotions can settle into our bodies and manifest physical symptoms. What thoughts and feelings do you have that are toxic to your health and well-being? Do you feel depressed and overwhelmed by the amount of stuff around you? Is your life filled with incompletion, both in work and relationships?

Take a look at your environment, and you will get a clear picture of where you are mentally and spiritually. If there's a lot of clutter in your environment, chances are you need an emotional detox, as well. Your physical clutter has an emotional toll. It can cause negative self-talk and can leave you stuck in self-defeating mental and emotional patterns. By clearing out the physical clutter, you begin the process of clearing the mental and emotional clutter.

Your Current Relationships

As we grow and change, so will our relationships. Just like reviewing your financial statements each year to see how you are doing and what to adjust for the following year, cleaning house may be necessary in your relationships to allow you to grow to who you want to be.

The first clue if you need to clean house would be how you feel when you are with some of the people in your life. Does hanging out with them give you energy? Do you feel positive, uplifted, and inspired when you around them? If this *is* the case, I would vote you stay connected to these kinds of people. However, if you feel sad, negative, drained, pulled into complaining, and fear, the energy of those people might be toxic for you. This will not help manifest a good relationship with your body or with a partner.

Think about how you experience different kinds of energy on a regular basis. Have you had the experience of being in a room full of people that are happy, upbeat, and positive and noticed that your mood was elevated by being around them? The energy level is high and can help bring you up to that level. For me, being around like-minded people that believe in a higher calling, want to change the world, and come from love, not fear, always lifts my mood. I walk away feeling that my energy tank has been filled up, and I am ready to conquer the world.

The opposite side of that is when you are in a good mood and walk into a room full of negative, angry, and sarcastic people. You can pretty much guarantee that over time the dominant energy in the room will start to wear on you and bring you down, even if you try to stay positive. You might walk away feeling frustrated and *icky* and not really know why. This negative energy may even affect your mood and attitude for the rest of the week. Energy is powerful; love and fear are both energy. You may not be able to see them, but you know they exist, and they influence what happens in your body, relationships, and life.

Make a list of all the people in your life and note whether they are a positive or negative influence over your life. Without blaming them for how you feel, notice if they have healthy, positive attitudes and habits in their own life, and how they treat you. Are they a complainer, and do they quickly negatively judge those around them? Are they calm, peaceful, and positive? This is a hard exercise because of all the potential history you may have with each person. Sleep on this one; choosing who you surround yourself with will affect you on every level.

Give yourself permission to throw things away, spend less time with negative people, cleanse your body and your mind. The more you get rid of, the lighter you will feel, the clearer you will think, and the more energized you will be. Clearing away the clutter allows you to see what has been hidden and what needs to be attended to in your life. When you remove clutter, you create space and you have the opportunity to start again. When you clean the slate, you are sending a message to the universe that you are ready to receive. You are receptive to the flow of life, to new ideas, to new gifts, to new experiences, and new relationships. You need to let go to receive. In the process, you will know that letting go is freedom. Trust that the universe will provide what you need, when you need it.

Chapter 5

Step 2: Sexual Fitness

"One is not born a woman, one becomes one." Simone de Beauvoir

We're going to talk about sexual fitness in a few different ways: the physical aspect, your sexual essence, and emotional well-being. My definition of sexual fitness is *the state or condition of being sexually, emotionally, and physically fit as the result of exercise, proper nutrition, and spiritual alignment.* The first thing that probably comes to mind is the physical aspect of fitness when it comes to sex. Do you have stamina? Are you flexible? Do you have the strength to contort your body and hold it in an uncommon position for a length of time? Are you happy in your body? We have to address your fitness and physical body first.

The Physical Aspect

The act of lovemaking is physical, and your fitness level affects your sexual performance. Stamina, strength, and confidence are required for a pleasurable experience. Sex can be like gymnastics: you may be requested to hold a position that challenges your body in ways your workout does not. What are the key elements to include in your workout to get the full potential of your physical body? For a free guide and more in depth descriptions of all the exercises, visit fit2love. info/exercises.

Cardio: Endurance training is necessary. The latest trend is to abandon steady state endurance training and only do interval training, but I disagree with that principle. Every type of exercise has a purpose. Unless you want to be a one-pump chump, you will want to be able to keep up for a long duration, and steady state endurance training is the way to go. Aim for at least 30 minutes of moderate intense exercise; this does not mean walking. Walking, while great for beginners, is not going to increase your overall fitness level, let alone your sexual fitness level. Try a ½ hour, 3 times a week, at a level 8 of intensity on a scale of 1-10. If you need to start at a lower level of intensity, work your way up. Hiking is also a great choice and can be enjoyed with others.

Upper body: Since lovemaking rarely resembles lifting weights in the gym, try doing isometric exercises to strength your ability to hold yourself up with your arms. An isometric exercise is where you hold a position in the exercise without doing the full range of motion. A plank, which is the starting position of a pushup where you just hold your upper body off the floor, is a great place to start to build endurance in your arms. If you are on top, you might need this strength. For beginners, focus on doing upper body exercises once a week and progress to two after a month. Intermediate and advanced exercisers need to add more isometrics to your routine and increase the intensity.

Leg Exercises: Squats, lunges, and leg presses are great choices for building thigh (quadriceps) and butt (gluteus maximus) strength: alternate isometric exercises with long *regular* sets of at least 30 repetitions. An isometric example for legs would be a wall-sit, not for anyone with knee problems. Use the example as a picture in your mind to understand the concept of isometrics. For example, you could do a set of squats for 30 repetitions very slowly (the set should be between 60-90 seconds total time), rest, and then hold a squat without moving for 60-90 seconds. The goal is to be able to hold yourself up while there is resistance on your body. You could also do this same example of alternating same muscle group exercises with a lunge. Execute 30 reps of a stationary lunge on each side and then hold a lunge for 60-90 seconds on each side. You will build muscle, strength, and endurance. Aim to do legs at least twice a week.

Hip Exercises: In order to gain flexibility in your hips, you need to do exercises in all active range of motion for your hips. Do not stretch because it does not create strength. Instead, do some Pilates exercises that challenge your hips, working both the inner thigh and outer hip. A few examples of these Pilates exercises are leg circles, frog, bow and arrow, sidekicks thread the needle, hot potato, side split, and skating. Visit fit2love.info/exercises for a full description of some of these exercises or find a Pilates studio near you.

Core Exercises: Thrusting your pelvis requires your abs to be strong enough to help do the job. The lower back muscles also need strength and flexibility to pull the pelvis back and maintain a contraction, if necessary. Exercises to concentrate on would be a full crunch, half crunch lower, bicycle, Pilates single leg pull, ball pass, spinal extension, and crunches on the ball to start. You want to have free flowing range of motion with your pelvis from front to back, as well as side to side. Do 2 to 3 sets of 30-40 reps to build endurance in these muscles to make lovemaking more physically enjoyable. These exercises can be found on the *30 Day JUMP Start Program* that you can download for free at invisiblefitness.com.

Internal: Doing kegels will strengthen the inner vaginal walls and help with orgasms for you and your partner. Kegels for men will help keep the prostate healthy. Keeping these muscles strong will also keep your sexual fitness youthful as you age.

Your Sexual Essence

Being sexually fit also means activating ecstasy, passion, and sensuality on a regular basis. This kind of energy is a magnet, not only for men, but for everyone around you. There is no need for a partner to exercise this aspect because it is an inside job. Every person is some part masculine and some part feminine. My guess is that I am 70% feminine and 30% masculine. I have fallen into the trap of activating my masculine energy more often and tipping the scale in reverse, because my career requires me to be productive, efficient, and goal oriented. These are masculine traits.

This became a problem when I was dating and looking for my man. I would treat it as a *job*, so I would go out on the town with focus and determination! Since I was activating my masculine energy, I would attract more feminine men, and that was not what I wanted. My good friend and acupuncturist, Shaheed, had to point it out to me. He said, "JJ, when you go out, take the badge off and put the gun down." I started to laugh because it became really clear to me how my energy was not inviting men to me, but repelling them. In order for me to attract a masculine man, I needed to live in my feminine more often.

This takes some practice in today's fast-paced, work-driven world, and it is not talked about openly. Women have strived to be like men for so long in the work environment that we don't recognize the damage it has done to our relationships. Unfortunately too often, we blame it on the men, when in reality, we have made the shift. I was fortunate enough to discover this information through a few workshops I had attended. Learning about and tapping into my feminine is what created the space to allow my husband to come forth. I don't know if our relationship would have worked had I taken the lead and used my masculine energy in the beginning. My spiritual path provided me with the lessons I needed to learn, and I took them very seriously.

One of the most effective tools I used to evoke my feminine was dancing. I started dancing when I was three years old, and it has always been a passion of mine. I didn't just do any kind of dancing, I did partner dancing—Salsa. In partner dancing, the woman has to learn to *let go and follow* so the man can lead. This concept is so powerful that it transformed my relationships instantly. I could truly tap into the feminine because I was trusting my partner and allowing him to lead me. My heart broke open and the wall of masculine melted as I learned to let go and follow. My brain got to shut down and my body took over. The freedom you get from allowing yourself to be in that space will make any woman glow with feminine energy. This is one example of how to practice inviting the feminine energy forth in your daily life.

Providing self pleasure in many forms will also help to activate your feminine energy of receiving. In fact, I would recommend self pleasure over settling for an interaction with someone less qualified to be your partner. When you honor your body, you attract someone who will also honor your body. Reminding yourself of your feminine gifts can create and maintain your sexual energy balance between masculine and feminine.

Emotional Well-being

This is the hardest part of sexual fitness because of the emotional baggage we all carry around about our bodies and the level of expectation we have about what we *should* look like. I was not immune to this, and working through it has been a lifelong process.

When I was in third, fourth, and fifth grade, I had bigger hips than the rest of the girls in the class. I figured out early on that I was never going to have the small, skinny frame that a lot of the girls I wanted to be like had. Breasts and hormones developed on me earlier than other girls; these were genetic facts of my body. You have genetic facts of your body, and the first step you have to do is accept them. *What you resist—persists.* The first step to changing what you have is to accept it.

Many people have unrealistic expectations of what is possible and what they are willing to do to achieve the body they want. Commonly, I hear a couch potato who hasn't exercised in years want to have the lean, toned, and perfect swimsuit model body. "I want to have a six pack. I want to be less than 18% body fat, have more energy, and I want it all in six months." Health and fitness are a habit, not an event. There is a progression to changing your body, and it will take time if you want it to last.

I am a trainer; therefore, most people think that means that I should want to be the leanest, most ripped, muscle-bound person I could be. I have struggled with that for years. Working in a gym, learning about resistance training, and seeing what the body is capable of makes anyone say, *wow, that would be really great to have, I would really love that.* Whether or not it is realistic or truly what is needed is another story. There are a lot of people who say they would like to be millionaires, but rarely do they take the action required to achieve it.

Back in 2000 when I was living in New York City, my roommate and I had a competition. A trainer, as well, he wanted to do a three-month program to see what he could do with his body in twelve weeks. At first, I wasn't interested, but as the day got closer, I thought, *I am going to prove I am a better trainer. I am going to go through everything I tell my clients to go through.*

Within the first seven weeks, I had lost 10 pounds and 7% body fat. He lost only 5 pounds and 2% body fat. I was feeling pretty successful in the first half of the program. What I noticed after the first 7 weeks was that I stopped trying so hard. Over the next 3 weeks, I only lost 3 pounds and no more body fat because in my mind I had already won—I was the better trainer.

Why didn't I challenge myself for the last five weeks? Mostly because I didn't want to; I didn't see the point. I had heard the stories of body builders and competitors living in the gym for hours and sucking on ice cubes before competitions. *There is no way in hell I am going to do that. Why do I have to put myself through that? Who am I trying to please?* Who are you trying to please?

I like the way I look. Would I like to be a little bit leaner? Sure. Would I like to build a little more muscle? Sure. Am I willing to do the work? Not right now because I am happy with where I am. What kind of body are you willing to work for and continue to do the work to keep? And why are you doing it? If you were to find your perfect mate who loves you exactly the way you are in the body you are in right now, would you still want to change? If you want to be accepted by someone else, you have to accept yourself first. Your workouts need to come from the place of self-love and respect, not fear and discontent. Wanting a strong, healthy body that performs well is the loving approach to your exercise routine.

Overcoming emotional hurdles can take some time, but you have the opportunity everyday to decide to love and accept yourself exactly the way you are as you start your new fitness and self-care program. My *6 Week Beach Body Program* is designed to help you reprogram your mind with ease by using hypnosis and creative visualizations so you can stop battling feelings of hatred and disgust toward your body. You can sample some of the tools we use for free, visit 6weekbeachbody.com/F2L.

Chapter 6

Step 3: A Food Love Affair

"One cannot think well, love well, sleep well, if one has not dined well." Virginia Woolf

We have lost touch with our relationship to food. With at least three opportunities every day to practice receiving the transfer of energy from our meals to our cells, eating has become a source of confusion and conflict, rather than a delightful pleasure. The lack of respect and abuse of food is one of the reasons why our health, as a culture, is rapidly declining. For some of us, the concept of doing anything except ordering in or going out seems like too much work. Our lives are too busy to slow down and prepare a home-cooked meal. Having a food love affair means having a deep, meaningful, respectful, and loving relationship to the food we put in our bodies.

In cultures throughout history, hunting, gathering, raising, and preparing foods was an honored and respected daily ritual. People were in tune with the abundance of each season and the different foods the earth provided throughout the year. Modern living has taken away the need of our attention to this. If you are looking for love, practice these principles with your food first. You have to create a love affair with food to attract the respect of your body and have success with health and weight management. To heal the obsession of dieting and calorie counting, you are going to treat food as your new lover, with whom you see the potential for a committed relationship. Rather than making food the enemy, you want to fall in love with food.

The Courtship

When you meet a man who interests you, the curiosity can be overwhelming. You want to know so many things: *Who he is? Where he is from? What does he do for a living? How was he raised?* Passion and excitement surround the quest for knowledge about this new person. It is an important step in finding the right partner. I want you to take a similar heightened interest in what you eat. Every day you fill your body with ingredients that make a huge impact on your health, state of mind, emotional well-being, and size of your waist. Take a look inside your refrigerator and kitchen cupboards and ask these questions: *How did this get made? How does it affect my body? Where did it come from?* Start to be more curious about seeking knowledge of the most vital relationship you already have—your diet. We take for granted what we consume everyday and how it impacts our lives. We are missing the spiritual connection to food.

Imagine you are looking at a red pepper. *How does it affect your body? How was it grown? Did the farmers use pesticides on the plants? Was it just picked, or has it been sitting in a grocery store for a few weeks after being shipped from a warehouse? What's the difference?* I chose the red pepper because my husband and I have just started growing our own vegetables, and we have green and red bell peppers. Prior to planting a garden, we were regularly shopping at the local farmer's market. At the last minute while preparing brunch for guests, I had the direct experience of comparing the shelf life of farm fresh veggies over the grocery store bought version. The store bought celery started to turn brown after two days, while the farmer's market celery lasted for over two weeks. This confirmed my choice to go directly to the farmers to get my produce as often as possible.

The red bell pepper has many nutrients you want to know about. Studies have shown that red bell peppers have significantly higher levels of nutrients than green. Red bell peppers contain lycopene, which helps to protect against cancer and heart disease. They are a good source of vitamin C, vitamin B6, beta carotene, and folic acid. Peppers contain a large amount of phytochemicals that act as antioxidants to protect against cataracts, blood clot formation, and reduce the risk of heart attacks and strokes. Sounds good, yes?

Can you get more excited about eating a red bell pepper and all the wonderful things it can help your body do? If you find yourself more interested in the red pepper, this is good news. You are creating a love affair with food.

The Engagement

Once you have decided to commit to changing your relationship with food, there are some adjustments you can make in your life. In a relationship with a person, you might decide to move in together and combine your belongings. You may open a bank account or add each other to your life insurance policies. By making a decision to engage more vegetables, you can plant a garden, make regular visits to the local farmer's market, or get home-delivered vegetables from the farm where available. When we moved into our house, my husband and I decided that we would plant a garden. Our love affair with vegetables took on a whole new level because we helped to prepare the soil, plant the seeds, give them water, and witnessed the vegetables grow. We gave it our energy, excitement, and nourished it with love. How exciting it was to be able to go out to the yard, pick the pepper to wash, clean, cut, and use in a meal with friends! My husband mentioned how nice of an experience it was to be able to pick the tomatoes off the vine for our dinner salads. Because we have a small yard, we purchased a composting box so we could contribute to creating more nutrient-dense soil for our vegetables. These are some examples of engaging your food and preparing for a lifetime together.

The Marriage

When you say "I do," you commit yourself to a lifetime with another person. In this lifetime, you may experience a series of highs and lows and everything in between. All relationships take work, and the one you have with your food is no different. Just like in a marriage, how you manage your relationship is what makes the difference between a healthy or unhealthy union. While growing up, most of my meals were homemade and homegrown; we rarely ate out. It became part of my life to pick vegetables out of the garden with my father and help prepare a meal with my mother. It set the foundation for my respect of food. Even though I strayed to processed and fast foods for a short period of time, I found my way back after gaining some weight and wanting to feel better in my body. I chose to commit myself to a love affair with food, and I am happy to say it's been happily ever after!

Until you face the relationship you have with your food, most of your health and body issues will not shift. Until you can appreciate the food that goes in your mouth, the effect it has on your body, and treat it with honor and respect, you may be forever a slave to diets and a negative body image. Imagine a calm, peaceful, sacred experience with food. Pick it, clean it, cut it, cook it, bless it, and savor it. Thank it for nourishing your body and keeping it strong and vibrant.

Food as Sex

Many foods are considered aphrodisiacs and have a strong power over the libido. Mineral and vitamin rich, most of these foods are low in fat and often appear in the shape of sexual organs they influence. Take your love affair with food to a whole new level by using its magic to increase the activity in the bedroom, as well as activate the sexual energy inside you. Martha Hopkins, author of *Inter Courses, An Aphrodisiac Cookbook,* provides history and recipes to help stimulate the dining experience for these tantalizing delectables.

Artichokes:	Like a blossom of a woman, needs the petals to be pulled back, slowly uncovering the treasure inside.
Asparagus:	Packed with potassium, phosperous, calcium and vitamin E. Keeps urinary track and hormone production healthy.
Avocado:	Cut in half, mimics the curves of woman. Aztec culture considered it powerful, and it melts in the mouth upon contact.

Basil: Alluring fragrance has been used for centuries to
                      keep wandering eyes focused at home.

Black Beans: Folklore says they increase fertility, like the bean
                      in the pod represents.

Chiles: Increases metabolism: gets blood rushing and
                      heart pumping.

Chocolate: Contains pheylethylamine, which is the same
                      molecule detected in our veins when we are in
                      love.

Figs: Layers of texture, sweet inside, and cuts like
                      butter.

Grapes: From wine, jam, and juice to art and the simple
                      grape, they are considered important for the
                      beauty and enhancement of many things, in
                      addition to their taste.

Honey: Honey encompasses sensuality and has been
                      connected with love and sex since the beginning
                      of time. Made from the nectar of flowers.

Oysters: Loaded with zinc, which helps with testosterone
                      production and increases libido in both men and
                      women.

Rosemary: Intoxicating aroma from a potent herb that
                      tickles your skin as you brush against it.

Strawberries: Mixture of tart and sweet, easy to hold and
                      enjoyable to the lips plain or dipped in chocolate.

Food as Health

Eating is our first basic need, and *you are what you eat* can be proven true. Beyond nutrition, most whole foods provide extra benefits. Here's a list of the properties commonly associated with a few familiar foods that you can start to incorporate into your diet.

Vegetables

Artichokes
- Aids digestion
- Lowers cholesterol
- Protects the heart
- Stabilizes blood sugar
- Guards against liver disease

Beets
- Controls blood pressure
- Combats cancer
- Strengthens bones
- Protects the heart
- Helps weight loss

Broccoli
- Strengthens bones
- Saves eyesight
- Combats cancer
- Protects the heart
- Controls blood pressure

Cabbage
- Combats cancer
- Prevents constipation
- Promotes weight loss
- Protects the heart
- Helps hemorrhoids

Carrots
- Saves eyesight
- Protects the heart
- Prevents constipation
- Combats cancer
- Promotes weight loss

Cauliflower
- Protects against prostate cancer
- Combats breast cancer
- Strengthens bones
- Banishes bruises
- Guards against heart disease

Chili Peppers
- Aids digestion
- Soothes sore throat
- Clears sinuses
- Combats cancer
- Boosts immune system

Garlic
- Lowers cholesterol
- Controls blood pressure
- Combats cancer
- Kills bacteria
- Fights fungus

Mushrooms
- Controls blood pressure
- Lowers cholesterol
- Kills bacteria
- Combats cancer
- Strengthens bones

Onions
- Reduces risk of heart attack
- Combats cancer
- Kills bacteria
- Lowers cholesterol
- Fights fungus

Sweet Potatoes
- Saves the eyesight
- Lifts mood
- Combats cancer
- Strengthens bones

Tomatoes
- Protects prostate
- Combats cancer
- Lowers cholesterol
- Protects the heart

Fruit

Apples
- Protects the heart
- Prevents constipation
- Blocks diarrhea
- Improves lung capacity
- Cushions joints

Apricots
- Combats cancer
- Controls blood pressure
- Saves the eyesight
- Shields against Alzheimer's
- Slows aging process

Bananas
- Protects the heart
- Quiets a cough
- Strengthens bones
- Controls blood pressure
- Blocks diarrhea

Blueberries
- Combats cancer
- Protects the heart
- Stabilizes blood sugar
- Boosts memory
- Prevents constipation

Cantaloupe
- Saves eyesight
- Controls blood pressure
- Lowers cholesterol
- Combats cancer
- Supports immune system

Cherries
- Protects the heart
- Combats cancer
- Ends insomnia
- Slows aging process
- Shields against Alzheimer's

Figs
- Promotes weight loss
- Helps stop strokes
- Lowers cholesterol
- Combats cancer
- Controls blood pressure

Grapefruit
- Protects against heart attacks
- Promotes weight loss
- Helps stop strokes
- Combats prostate cancer
- Lowers cholesterol

Grapes
- Saves eyesight
- Conquers kidney stones
- Combats cancer
- Enhances blood flow
- Protects the heart

Lemons
- Combats cancer
- Protects the heart
- Controls blood pressure
- Smoothes skin
- Stops scurvy

Limes
- Combats cancer
- Protects the heart
- Controls blood pressure
- Smoothes skin
- Stops scurvy

Mangoes
- Combats cancer
- Boosts memory
- Regulates thyroid
- Aids digestion
- Shields against Alzheimer's

Oranges
- Supports immune systems
- Combats cancer
- Protects the heart
- Straightens respiration

Peaches
- Prevents constipation
- Combats cancer
- Helps stop strokes
- Aids digestion
- Helps hemorrhoids

Pineapple
- Strengthens bones
- Relieves colds
- Aids digestion
- Dissolves warts
- Blocks diarrhea

Prunes
- Slows aging process
- Prevents constipation
- Boosts memory
- Lowers cholesterol
- Protects against heart disease

Strawberries
- Combats cancer
- Protects the heart
- Boosts memory
- Calms stress

Watermelon
- Protects prostate
- Promotes weight loss
- Lowers cholesterol
- Helps stop strokes
- Controls blood pressure

Dairy

Yogurt
- Guards against ulcers
- Strengthens bones
- Lowers cholesterol
- Supports immune systems
- Aids digestion

Grains & Legumes

Beans
- Prevents constipation
- Helps hemorrhoids
- Lowers cholesterol
- Combats cancer
- Stabilizes blood sugar

Oats
- Lowers cholesterol
- Combats cancer
- Battles diabetes
- Prevents constipation
- Smoothes skin

Rice
- Protects the heart
- Battles diabetes
- Conquers kidney stones
- Combats cancer
- Helps stop strokes

Fats

Avocados
- Battles diabetes
- Lowers cholesterol
- Helps stop strokes
- Controls blood pressure
- Smoothes skin

Chestnuts
- Promotes weight loss
- Protects the heart
- Lowers cholesterol
- Combats cancer
- Controls blood pressure

Flax
- Aids digestion
- Battles diabetes
- Protects the heart
- Improves mental health
- Boosts immune system

Olive Oil
- Protects the heart
- Promotes weight loss
- Combats cancer
- Battles diabetes
- Smoothes skin

Walnuts
- Lowers cholesterol
- Combats cancer
- Boosts memory
- Lifts mood
- Protects against heart disease

Honey
- Heals wounds
- Aids digestion
- Guards against ulcers
- Increases energy
- Fights allergies

Drinks & Condiments

Water
- Promotes weight loss
- Combats cancer
- Conquers kidney stones
- Smoothes skin

Green Tea
- Combats cancer
- Protects the heart
- Helps stop strokes
- Promotes weight loss
- Kills bacteria

Savoring Your Love Affair

Food is nourishment, as well as pleasure. You wouldn't rush through a date with the person you love, so treat your dining experience as sacred. Slowing down and enjoying what is on your plate means chewing it thoroughly, savoring the flavors, textures and pleasures of each bite. By slowing down when you eat, you will experience the food with more satisfaction and need less of it. Practice your love affair with food every day, and you will transform your body, as well as your experience.

Chapter 7

Step 4: Wear Sexy Underwear

"Sex appeal is 50% what you've got and 50% what people think you've got." Sophia Loren

In 2004, I attended a self-growth camp where we were challenged to our limits physically, mentally, and emotionally every day. On the third day, I was chosen out of the crowd in my camp to have a public *reading* by the instructor. I watched him read a few others before me and thought, *How the hell can he say those kinds of things about them? He doesn't even know anything about them!*

The comments were very direct and often evoked tears from the other women. He was not being mean or disrespectful; the statements were just brutally honest and often not easy to hear. When it was my turn, I put on my best poker face and prepared myself. He only asked me one question.

"Are you single?"

"Yes. Well, I just got out a relationship, but I am not sure that it is really over," I replied.

He knew nothing else about me, yet he proceeded to describe me very accurately.

"You are using your mind too much. You use your intellect and try to compete with the men, instead of using your feminine gifts to lure them. Embrace your feminine energy, and it will help to you flow more easily through all parts of your life. Stop pushing."

I was blown away.

My friend Michelle's mouth dropped to the floor because of how precise his statements were about who I was and what I needed to do. The instructor appointed Michelle my accountability partner for my homework, which was to buy sexy pink lingerie and dance around in it every day before I started the day—everyday.

Did I do it? Yes. I performed this ritual for about a week until I decided it was too forced for me to do it every day by myself. To make this work, I needed to find a way to make it something I enjoyed doing. The point of the exercise was to adorn myself and activate the feminine energy within me through music and dance. Being a salsa dancer, I already had it built into my life, so I applied the principle to my evenings out to dance. The hot salsa club to go to on Saturday nights had a dress code, so I used this as my excuse to break out the sexy dresses, the shiny jewelry, and add some glitter to my evening makeup. I had no other place in my life where dressing like this was acceptable and celebrated.

I understood the message but decided to translate it into my life in a way that supported my regular practice. The bottom line for most of us is to activate our feminine energy and stop pushing so much. When I met my husband, I was consistently dancing three to four times a week and having a blast. My feminine energy was very alive in me, which helped me evoke his masculine energy and attention.

Dancing around my house in my sexy underwear wasn't a problem; it just was not as fun as dancing at the clubs. I wanted to find a practice I would do often without resistance. For some women, wearing sexy underwear is all it takes to easily add this energy into their daily life.

Matching Bras and Panties

Here is a story from Veronica Rose, who thought it was a silly idea until she tried it:

I had a friend who was single and had a drawer full of lingerie. She said to me one day, "You don't wear lingerie for the men. You wear it because it makes you feel feminine. Pretty matching bras and panties remind you that you love yourself and you are important."

Before this, I thought it was a waste of money and you only did it for a man once you're married. After having a baby and struggling with the last few pounds of baby weight, I got to the point where I would try anything to make me feel better.

So I tried it. I ordered four sets.

That was the best thing I ever did, and I recommend it to all women. When you walk out the door, it's like dressing for success, only you're dressing for yourself underneath. Nobody else knows, but it doesn't matter because you are doing it for yourself. Your outside is dressed for success, but your inside is dressed for being the woman that you are; it adds that little zing to your energy. At least it did for me, and I felt better about myself.

If you need new lingerie, why not buy something that you like that's pretty and colorful? It doesn't even have to be colorful, if you can't wear that. For a long time, I wore a white uniform, so it had to be white lace.

Maybe it won't work for everybody, but figure out what makes you feel pretty, feminine, and sexy and then go from there. When you put it on and you go to work, you are the only one that knows what's under there, and you feel it. You should try it, and then you'll know what I'm talking about. Before you knock it, try it. It's not that expensive. Just buy one. I highly recommend it.

Get on the Dance Floor

As I have mentioned, dancing was my key to unlocking my feminine energy when I started learning partner dances like salsa. Not only is partner dancing a great place to practice letting go and giving up control, it's also a great place to meet other single men and women. Every dance class I went to was filled with all kinds of people wanting to learn how to dance. In the salsa world, dancing is like a sport. You expect to dance with multiple partners, and there are rules.

First, the woman is supposed to wait for a man to ask her to dance. Secondly, most of the time, you only dance one song with each man at a time if you do not know your partner. Unlike hip hop clubs, where agreeing to dance with a man might mean he will be following you around for the rest of the night; salsa is not like that. Once you start to make friends, you may choose to dance multiple songs with a partner, but saying no often is expected and practiced.

Women have total freedom to dress however they please—the more feminine and sexy, the better. My favorite lesson is that women are supposed to follow and not lead. I started teaching salsa a few years ago, and I loved to lead the women so I could point out how they are not really letting go. Most women want to be good students and do it right, so they learn the moves and perform them, whether or not they have been led to do so. Letting go means you are not the driver; many women struggle with allowing the man to lead them. I want to teach all women to feel the freedom of following. It's like having a chef, maid, driver, babysitter, and masseuse all in one—you feel like you are on a cloud.

Dancing has a great side benefit besides infusing women with feminine energy; it's great exercise. Once you find a dance you love, you can do it all night. Hours go by and you forget your life. The bubble of the dance world sucks you in, and next thing you know, you have burned 1,000 calories having the time of your life. There are all types of dance and music out there. If you are not ready for a class, dance in your sexy underwear at home to your favorite song.

Get a Stanford

In *Sex and the City*, Sarah Jessica Parker's character, Carrie Bradshaw, has something every single woman needs—a gay man. Besides her gal pals, Carrie's best bud is Stanford. The character of Charlotte also has her best guy pal, Anthony, to play with. They are the perfect date when its couple's only, and it's fun to have another friend interested in the same things you are!

I learned years ago that I wanted companionship over just intimacy. Having many gay friends, I found it easy to forget that I was single when I was in the company of a gay man. A man is still a man, and it's nice to have the masculine energy around, even if they have no interest in sleeping with you.

During the few months before Brian decided to come forth and ask me out, I already had found good company in my gay friends. We went to the movies, dancing, dinner, and stayed in to enjoy a homemade meal and a bottle of wine. I had all the things I wanted in a relationship except the sex, and I was perfectly okay with that because I had dancing and a few toys to take care of that.

Because I was happy, having a good time and feeling complete within myself, I sent out the message that I was doing just fine. Being happy and vibrant attracts others that want to play with you and be happy, too. The truth was that I was fine. I was having a blast.

Getting a Stanford is different than buying a handbag—people are not disposable. Find people you genuinely like and want to have in your life. Fulfill the companionship role in your life with someone you enjoy being around. Focus on having fun and being happy. It's that simple.

Buy Yourself Roses

The most universally recognized and beloved flower in the world is the rose. It represents love, affection, compassion, purity, innocence, and passion. For centuries, roses have been used all over the world as medicinal tonics to help cure ailments; rose flower essence supports and protects the heart from emotional pain and trauma. These beautiful flowers are commonly used as mood enhancers. It is customary in many parts of the world to give roses as a token of one's love, affection, and devotion. I am suggesting you give yourself a token of your love, affection, and devotion.

Having fresh flowers in your home raises the vibration around you. All plants have the ability to add energy to an environment, but bright colors and fragrant smells can elevate you even higher. Fresh flowers are hard not to notice and catching a glimpse of them every day can warm your heart. Each flower has its own personality and sends its own message. While red roses often signify deep love, white and pink roses are considered friendly. When I need a pick me up, I buy yellow daisies because they say *be happy* to me.

Wear Sexy Underwear is about doing something for yourself that makes you feel special, sexy, adored, and alive. Embodying this has many forms. Find a practice that evokes this energy for you and commit to it every week. Notice when your energy changes because the energy you attract will also change.

Chapter 8
Step 5: Thank Your Lucky Stars

"We can only be said to be alive in those moments when our hearts are conscious of our treasures." **Thornton Wilder**

Please understand that you are perfect just the way you are right now. The journey you are on is unique and special. There is nothing wrong or broken about you. Your mind and body are working perfectly even when they are doing things you don't like.

You get constant feedback from your body and emotions about where you are in the moment so you can decide where you want to go next. This is a spiritual journey, as much as a physical and emotional journey, of changing your body and manifesting love from within, as well as from another.

While there are many factors in life that are out of your control, you do have the ability to manage your thoughts and how you react to every situation. How you perceive your experiences will color the kinds of emotions attached to them. Choosing a more positive and hopeful outlook will produce better feelings. There are always two points of view to choose from in every situation: what is working and what is not.

Focus on what is working to practice gratitude every single day. This will not only help you manifest more of what you want, it will also make you happy immediately. When you can control your thoughts and feelings, you influence your happiness. If you find this difficult to do or sustain on your own, talking to someone like a psychologist, counselor, or life coach can help you shift your thoughts and change your feelings. Start by thanking your lucky stars.

What is Gratitude?

*Gratitude is appreciation for people, places, and things, as well as,
for ideas, qualities, and feelings*
Gratitude is thankfulness, and I use it like a key
a key to inspire strangers, my friends, and me
a key to life that sets me free
a key to heal insult and injury
a key to awareness, when I refuse to dream
a key to finding forgiveness and feeling peace
a key to manifest my desires, what I want, and who I choose to be
a key to light the dark times, when I can't see
a key to expressing my preferences, what I love, the real me
a key to feeling the present moment, gently
a key to reconnect me to humility
*a key to boundless opportunity, when I get caught in my limited
certainty*
a key to transcendence, imagination, and epiphany
a key to turn the hardest moment into a glorious journey
a key to the only foolproof system of love in the galaxy
a key to access infinite possibilities
and when I share my gratitude, gratitude enriches you and me
*Gratitude is actually the doorway, **choice** is the real key*
The best part about gratitude is that gratitude
is always... absolutely... free!

"Gratitude is" by Macarena Luz Bianchi

Having Gratitude Can Positively Affect Your Future

Research has shown that people who think positively have an
increased capacity for happiness. Choosing to be grateful will support
your efforts of maintaining healthy habits, such as regular exercise
and a healthy diet. The connection between gratitude and health goes
back throughout history; philosophers and religious leaders have
proclaimed gratitude as a virtue that is integral to health and well-
being for centuries. Positive psychology is the current movement

of mental health professionals who are taking a close look at how gratitude can benefit our health. The Mayo Clinic staff reports that researchers continue to explore the effects of positive thinking and optimism on our bodies.

Health benefits from positive thinking:

- Increased life span

- Lower rates of depression

- Lower levels of stress

- Greater resistance to the common cold; better immunity

- Better psychological and physical well-being

- Reduced risk of death from cardiovascular disease

- Better coping skills during hardships and times of stress

Where to Start?

What we think and how we think are habits. We have practiced them over and over until they became second nature, which is why we feel justified when we have a negative reaction to something and call it natural. The best way to start to change these habits is by having a Gratitude Journal. I use one every night before I go to bed to make a list of what went well during the day. There are predesigned journals out there that you can buy, or you can simply use a notebook or piece of paper. The easiest way to start is by asking yourself what you are grateful for and make a list. This directs your attention to things that feel good. We often overlook these things because we have been trained to worry about what it is we did not accomplish each day. Focusing on things such as incomplete tasks can add stress to your body and emotions. Stress repels joy. You get to choose one.

Set a regular time aside in your mind everyday to make a gratitude list. I make mine before bed and keep the journal on the nightstand. This is a system that works for me. You may want to do it after dinner or when you get home from work to reframe your mind and focus on what positive things happened during your day. The important thing is to do it, regardless of the system you choose.

Body Facts to be Grateful For

To get you started, here are some amazing facts about the body that we take for granted:

- Your brain triples in size between birth and adulthood, until it weighs as much as the heart and lungs put together.
- We are about 70 percent water.
- We give birth to 100 billion red cells every day.
- In relation to body size, the human brain is larger than the brain of any animal on earth.
- Our blood is on a 60,000-mile journey.
- Our heart beats around 100,000 times every day.
- Every minute your two kidneys, no larger than a fist, are hard at work filtering waste products and excess water from your blood.
- The average adult's skin spread out flat is large enough to cover a room 9 feet by 15 feet.
- We exercise at least 30 muscles when we smile.
- In an average lifetime of 70 years, a person sheds 441 lbs. of skin.
- The average red blood cell lives for 120 days.
- A baby grows from a dot-sized fertilized egg into a fully developing baby in the space of just 40 weeks.
- Our nose is our personal air-conditioning system: it warms cold air, cools hot air, and filters impurities.
- We are born with all of our organs in full working order. For most of us, despite the abuse we dish out to our bodies, they will last largely unaided until our dying day. By then, they will have performed some incredible feats.
- There are more living organisms on the skin of a single

human being than there are human beings on the surface of the Earth.

- Your lungs will have inhaled and exhaled enough air to fill either 1 of the 2 largest airships ever built 1.5 times over.
- Your body has about 5.6 liters or 6 quarts of blood that circulates through the body three times every minute.
- Your heart will have beaten more than 2.5 billion times, pumping enough blood around the body to fill the fuel tanks of 700 jumbo jets.
- The human body can function without a brain.
- Your eyeballs are 3.5% salt.
- Your stomach and intestines will have digested the weight of six bull African elephants or more in food.

There are hundreds of facts about the body that we could focus on at any given moment to shift from a state of frustration to gratitude. Reading this list every day can also help you appreciate the body you were given. If you get stuck, start your gratitude list every night with one of these facts to set the mood.

Thank your lucky stars by making a gratitude list for every aspect of your life: work, family, and friends. As stated in the movie *Kung Fu Panda* by Master Oogway, the master tortoise of the Jade Palace, "You are too concerned about what was and what will be. There is a saying: yesterday is history, tomorrow is a mystery, but today is a gift. That is why it is called the *present*." Learn to be in the moment and enjoy the gift of the present you have right now.

Chapter 9

Putting Yourself First

"Love yourself first and everything else falls into line. You really have to love yourself to get anything done in this world." Lucille Ball

Jody Lay is President, General Manager, and a partner of Hansen Engineering Company. Hansen Engineering is a manufacturer of precision aircraft parts and has recently attained a Preferred Supplier status of Silver for all divisions of Boeing. Hansen is an approved supplier for Spirit Aerosystems on the 737 Next-Generation aircraft program, and they have 39,000 sq. ft. of manufacturing and office space in Los Angeles, California. Jody Lay is responsible for coordinating and overseeing all phases of production. He has been one of my clients since 2008 and was the first person I thought of when creating *Fit 2 Love*.

JJ: When we met, you had embarked on a new life-changing program. You had committed yourself to a lot of different health-related journeys under the care of a doctor, nutritionist, and with me as your fitness trainer. Tell us a little bit about who you are.

Jody: I'm 59 years old. I'm in the machine shop business, and we mostly build airplane parts. I have 53 employees working for me, which can be very stressful at times, and have spent the last 30 years working behind a desk. During this time, I gained a lot of weight and became increasingly unhealthy. I noticed I was tired all the time. I was also in a relationship that I wasn't really happy with, so I needed to make some major changes.

JJ: What was the state of your health and wellness? On a scale of one to ten, ten being the best you can be, how well did you take care of yourself? Had you been working out before we met?

Jody: Oh, not very well, like a three or four. I have always worked out, water-skied and snow skied. I had recently taken up a new sport called hydrofoiling. This sport is not as tough on my body as waterskiing, but it's a lot more fun. But like my snow skiing, it was all starting to take a toll on me. I was pretty heavy. At one point, I think I reached 276 pounds, and I'm 6'2". I'd go out and maybe ski half a day: get there at nine and be done by noon. I would be tired and beat, and my friends would continue skiing the rest of the day, so I felt kind of left out.

        After working with you, JJ, I found out that a lot of what I was doing in my workouts was not effective and a big waste of time. Even though I worked out five days a week, I was not losing weight. You changed all of that.

JJ: What pushed you to want to get to the next level?

Jody: One of the things that kind of pushed me was the girl I was dating said that she knew I was always dieting and trying to lose weight and never really succeeding. I'd lose 5 or 10 pounds. Then, I'd put it back on. She mentioned maybe I should have that bariatric surgery: gastric bypass. I said to myself, *I want to lose weight, but I don't want to have surgery.* Browsing through a magazine one day, I saw an old guy who was 57 years old sitting in a boat with a big gut, and he reminded me of myself. Except, there was also a picture of him ten years later at 67 years old, but he looked like he was 30. He had the body of a 30 year old! Not an ounce of fat on him; he was strong and muscular. He looked like he was in really great shape. It was obvious that the picture was real; it didn't seem like it was a touched up or altered in anyway. That picture is what did it for me.

JJ: And before the journey started, you were in a relationship. How was that going?

Jody: It was a very difficult relationship. I wasn't happy with her. She wasn't happy with me. We were together, but it wasn't really very good. We did the best we could, but neither one of us was really happy with each other.

JJ: You were emotionally unhappy about your health, body, and current relationship. You then made a huge commitment to make some major changes in all aspects of your life. I had suggested that you do a detox for your body to clean the slate and get focused. It was a nice surprise to see you not just detoxing your body with food and adding more exercise, you also "cleaned house" with your relationship. It put you in a new space. Witnessing your transition is one of the reasons why we're having this interview. In fact, you were the first person I thought of when first creating *Fit 2 Love.*

You took yourself to another level of self-care and attended to the things that mattered in your life. There was a certain point at which enough was enough and you wanted more— you wanted better. You didn't want to struggle with your relationship and body and wanted the pieces to fit better than they did.

Jody: They never did fit.

JJ: Right. There was a certain point in which you started paying more attention to the state of your well-being and your level of happiness. Your bad relationship was a stress factor in your life, which also affected your health. You ended that relationship so that you could release all the stress and drama and focus on things that made you feel good.

Jody: You are absolutely right. We have talked about this, and you're absolutely right.

JJ: Leaving that relationship was an act of self-love. It was being able to accept: This isn't working. Many people are afraid of being alone, so they stay in bad relationships. Internally, you were probably thinking that you deserve to be in a better place, whether it is with someone or alone. It was time to step up and feel better on every level.

Jody: Yep. I haven't really consciously thought a lot about those things, but it's exactly what happened.

JJ: Now, you were in this space where it was all about you. What do I want? What do I need? What am I going to do? In this transition, you spent more time taking care of you and doing things that were fun and exciting by yourself. You booked a trip to Cabo almost immediately after your break up and took a trip to the river to hydrofoil with your friends for a week before that. You have always been very dedicated to having fun on a regular basis, and that is as important as exercise. I admire you for that and wished all my clients would play as often as you do!

        As you were totally consumed with having fun and being in a self-care space, you then accidently met the woman that you are now going to marry. What's different about her?

Jody: Lynda is a caregiver, like me, and she likes to take care of people. She is loving; she's got a great heart. She's somebody who I feel comfortable with. We like the same things. We like to work out and run together. On our first date, we went running.

JJ: On a scale of one to ten, after your breakup, how well were you taking care of yourself?

Jody: Maybe six or so. Now I feel like I'm at maybe an eight and ready to go to the next level again. I want to get to a nine or a ten. Our workouts are getting harder, and my diet's getting better. I've had a lot of stress at work lately and kind of fell back a little bit. But long term, I know I'm going to be fine. I'm going to continue to improve. I keep getting better and going to another level. And maybe, a year from now, or two years from now, I'll say, "You know what, I wasn't really at a six, I was only at a five, and then I was at a six or an eight." I'll have a new goal, a new level that I want to reach. I'll just have to reevaluate where those goals were. Because a year ago, I thought I was giving it everything. I know that I can give more.

JJ: Would you agree that the healthier you became, the more time you spent on taking care of *you* in all aspects, helped *you* to manifest and bring *you* the relationship *you* really wanted?

Jody: Yes. It's very, very true. I have become healthier and healthier, and my life has changed. I have a woman now who is very interested in what we eat and how we eat together. We still fight over some things. As far as where I was a year ago, I had broken up with my old girlfriend and just happened to meet this new girl. I wasn't really looking for it. In fact, my goal was to not meet anyone. It was actually to stay away from any women for at least six months. My goal was to work on myself, so I was working very hard. I was working with you, working out, running, and watching my diet. Then, along came Lynda. I wasn't looking for it. It just happened and made everything even better. It made all the working out more fun.

JJ: Were you also at the healthiest place you had been in a long time or ever?

Jody. In 30 years, I was at the healthiest place I had ever been.

JJ: What was interesting about Lynda that made her the marrying kind? What made her so special, wonderful, and different to you? What were you looking for in a woman?

Jody: I was not looking. She was living in Marietta, and I was in Orange County. We didn't get to see each other often: only on the weekends. We would go running on our dates. When she arrived, she wouldn't have any makeup on, and I'd be in my workout clothes. We never even really got to go out to dinner within the first month. Our dates were sweaty messes. After the workout, we'd have some breakfast and talk. I realized what a great person she was. It wasn't about style and fashion because I never saw her in regular clothes; she was always in workout clothes. It was just the two of us. We talked. We talked about what she had been doing. She was a single mother. She raised her two children nearly singlehandedly for the last 15 years and with very little support from her ex-husband. At the same time, she managed to go to college and get a degree. That's not very easy for a single woman who was also taking care of her 83-year-old father on top of raising her boys. She was not just taking care of herself, being healthy, and working out all the time, but she was taking care of her whole family. I hear her on the phone with her brother, and I am in awe. She was sort of the leader of the family. I'm sort of the leader of my family. It's not something we sought; it's just who we are. We had a lot in common that way.

JJ: There are women everywhere who think the number one thing a man's looking at is how well their body looks. Even though I know that men are visually oriented and that is going to be important, I want you to give women some advice about some of the other things that are important to men. What would you advise women to focus on?

Jody: I think they should focus on taking care of themselves mentally, taking care of their health, and not really worry about what the man thinks or what he's looking for. I think you're right. I was with a woman who only focused on how she looked. She didn't really care about anything else; she just wanted to be thin. She wanted to have her nails done all the time, and her hair and makeup had to be perfect. She had to dress very, very well. I wasn't happy with that woman. She was sort of narcissistic. It's not what I really want. I do want someone who cares about herself, but those superficial things are not important.

JJ: Lynda doesn't take care of herself because she cares what everybody else thinks?

Jody: No. She works out because she wants to work out. She wants to be healthy and likes the feeling of working out. It's not about what other people think. Lynda is beautiful, but it's not just what you see on the outside. It's her heart. It's her caring for other people. There's a lot more to her. She's substantial. She's not fluff. Does that make sense?

JJ: Sure. You found the person you were supposed to be with when you were taking the best care of yourself that you had in 30 years. This is valuable for single women to grasp. You've said that Lynda is substantial. She doesn't do things because she cares what other people think. She does them for herself. She has confidence, independence, strength, and beauty.

Jody: Yes. She also has a very, very tender heart. At first, she guarded it, but I saw it. I would get glimpses of it. She didn't show it to most people, and I knew it was there. Then, I did something that I have never done for anybody: I wrote her a poem about her tender heart.

JJ: Ah! Wow!

Jody: I'd never done that ever. It chokes me up right now thinking about it. She read it and cried because I saw something in her that she guarded. That's what I fell in love with. I want to share it with you.

> *I caught a glimpse of her heart today.*
> *She briefly let her mask down.*
> *And through the looking glass,*
> *I caught a glimpse of her soft and tender heart.*
> *Her vulnerable heart.*
> *And mine fluttered...*

JJ: That is so beautiful! Thank you for sharing that with all the women who dream about a man writing them a poem. That's amazing. She's a very lucky woman, and I know you feel like a lucky man.

Jody: I do. We had that conversation earlier this week when we realized we'd been together for a year, and we want to make it the rest of our lives. It's not always easy, but it's very, very good.

JJ: Is this the happiest time you can remember?

Jody: Yes, absolutely. I have never had a year go by faster that was
         more exciting and happy. I love her family. They're great; they
         can come over any time. She loves my family. My daughter
         was over last night, and we were all just hugging and laughing
         together. It was great.

JJ: For all the women out there who want to have the same kind of
         man in their life, what advice could you give them?

Jody: Be yourself. Whatever you're doing, do it for yourself. You have
         to take care of yourself first, and everything else will be fine.

JJ: Awesome.

Jody: I never really thought about it before, but I was taking care
         of myself, and I wasn't thinking about anyone else. I wasn't
         thinking about Lynda. I was thinking about taking care of
         myself because I had a lot of things I wanted to do. You know I
         don't sit around a lot.

JJ: No, you don't!

Jody: I met somebody who wants to do the same things I do. We want
         to travel. We want to be healthy. That's why we take care of
         ourselves. We want to have fun. We spent a week at the river
         hydrofoiling last month. The month before that, we were in
         Maui for five days. In a month, we're going to Cabo for a week.
         In March, we're going to Colorado skiing. You've got to take
         care of yourself if you want to enjoy those things. We both try
         really hard, but sometimes we fall down. Sometimes, we eat or
         drink too much, but we always get back up and start again. We
         always try to take care of ourselves.

JJ: You guys are doing great. Anything else you want to share?

Jody: I was taking care of myself. She was taking care of herself.
         Then, we just kind of ran into each other. It was easy.

JJ: Awesome. Thank you, Jody. I'm so excited. You were the first person I thought of for this project because I got to witness you live the concepts of *Fit 2 Love* and enjoyed watching your transformation.

Jody: Thank you.

Steps Jody Used to Attract the Love of His Life

Step 1: Clean the Slate. Jody started a total health makeover, completed a nine-day detox to clean his body, and ended a seven-year relationship to take time to concentrate on himself.

Step 3: A Food Love Affair. As part of the total health makeover, Jody eliminated gluten and dairy from his diet and added more fruits and vegetables. He also concentrated on smaller portions after completing the detoxification.

Step 5: Thank Your Lucky Stars: Jody is an upbeat and positive man who always looks for the best in people. He maintains many long-term friendships, as well as loyal, longstanding employees. Every session, Jody would look for evidence of his improvement and be grateful for making the commitment to his health. Repeatedly I would hear, "This is the best thing I have ever done for myself. I feel better than I ever have."

Loving yourself can be very simple when you attend to the things that make you happy. Jody learned by trial and error how to prioritize his self-care. He learned his lesson when he was ready, and it paid off! Once you practice honoring yourself first, it gets easier. Just like many busy, stressed out men and women out there, he learned how to balance it with his self-care when he was ready.

Chapter 10

Mending the Wounds

"Our first and last love is - self-love." **Christian Bovee**

Jennifer Torok is a wife and mother of two, who struggled since she was 12 with her weight, an eating disorder, and her self-image. She has done countless weight loss programs and therapy in search of a way to end the self-sabotaging cycle that was ruling her life. In the summer of 2009, Jennifer was a participant in my *6 Week Beach Body Program*, where I got to witness her daily journals and her self-love transformation.

JJ: Thanks for being here, Jen. Tell us about your history with fitness and your weight.

Jenny: Well, what program haven't I done, right? My dieting started when I was 12. I started dieting, counting calories, and looking at magazines for how to stay thin when I was 12. I was in theater and dance; my mother had an eating disorder, and it was just so much in my consciousness already. I was going through puberty, and my body was changing. I started to not feel good about who I was on the outside. My mind kept telling me, "You know, we're going to need to fix you."

JJ: How did you get the idea that you needed to be fixed?

Jenny: From the family I was born into. Who I was as a person made my family uncomfortable. I was very enthusiastic and excited about life. I was the lightning rod of the family. My parents were struggling with their own addictions, so their way of dealing with me was to act like "we've got to get this girl to shut up because we're having a hard time here, and she's too much for us." And then, I started binging when I was 16.

JJ: Can you talk about why you binged?

Jenny: I binged because life was hard for me. I couldn't deal with my emotions. I couldn't deal with my life. I couldn't deal with what I didn't like about my life. I grew up in an Italian family that loved food. Conversations and activities were so centered around food all the time. Food was the comfort and also the enemy; food was essentially my drug of choice. Our house was very strict about things like junk food. I'd go to my friend's house where they could have all the junk food they wanted; it represented freedom. I would go and binge on junk food because it was an act of rebellion against my family—my strict, rigid family with all their rules about food and body.

I think it truly became a chemical imbalance because I would get nervous if I thought I felt good. *I can't feel good. I can't possibly feel good.* I wasn't able to just let myself feel healthy. I would eat so I wouldn't feel good.

A big awakening happened after college because I started working. I got a full-time job teaching, woke up and said, "Okay, I've got to take care of this. This is ridiculous. It is really taking over too much of my life, and I feel hung over in the morning. My head is cloudy, and I don't feel good."

I started reading a lot about nutrition and trying to deal with the cravings. Then I got married and knew I wanted to get pregnant, so I had to really tackle this. I sat with a therapist and had never, until this point, considered that I had an eating disorder.

JJ: So at 28 years old, after having this behavior and all these feelings since you were 12, you turned around, looked back and said, "I have an eating disorder?"

Jenny: Yes. Exactly. You've got it.

JJ: Did this behavior feel normal to you? Were other people doing it around you?

Jenny: Yeah. Everybody was talking about dieting and calories. We would work hard all week, and then we'd go and drink and just eat a bunch on the weekend. Work hard, play hard. But I really ate to numb out. I was around all these other people who were numbing out, or at least trying to numb out, so it was just normal. This is what we did.

JJ: What were you numbing yourself from?

Jenny: I was numbing myself from my anger at my family of really feeling not supported and not loved. They didn't have my back. They were not there when I needed them in some pretty significant ways, and I felt abandoned.

JJ: Now were there ways in which you would behave or do things to get what felt like love from your parents?

Jenny: Oh, yeah. I would basically be overly dramatic. If I felt too good for too long, it was a scary because that meant I would be okay and they would not give me attention. The only way I could get attention was if I was in crisis. So I darned well better keep myself in crisis so I can have their attention; otherwise, forget it. They weren't interested in me if I was healthy. They were interested in my crisis. This continued until I was in my twenties, when I started doing work that really compelled me beyond the drama of my personal life. I needed to get a handle on it. *I'm an adult. It's time to really take responsibility for my health and my happiness.*JJ: Would you say that you were happy at all during this time?

| Jenny: | Oh, God, I was absolutely happy so much of the time. There was happiness. I wasn't a depressed person at all. I think most people would say that I was pretty happy. |

JJ: If you were happy, then how do you recognize the problem?

Jenny: I was happy, but not happy enough. I wasn't at peace because it was all conditional happiness. It was happiness contingent upon external things: the job was good, pay was good, boyfriend was good, and body was good. As long as all these external things were in place, I could be happy. But, if anything fell apart, forget it, my life was in crisis. It was not solid ground I was standing on.

JJ: How did you meet your husband?

Jenny: I met my husband in Portland, Oregon. I left my job and had moved from Washington DC to Portland, Oregon to be close to my family. I followed my gut with this one. I had a very strong sense that I needed to be with my family out West. My intention was to be close for the birth of my nephew, so I could be there when he was born. I thought it would be temporary. *I'll be here for a year.*

When I got to Portland, I immediately got a great job. I took the job, withdrew my teaching contract in DC, and within six months I had met Aaron. We met through a mutual friend at a time when I was seeing somebody else. Coincidentally, I had some psychic guy tell me I was going to meet my husband, and I thought, *whatever.* Then I met Aaron and thought, "Oh, my God. He was right. That's really freaky."

JJ: How quickly did you know when you met Aaron that you were going to marry him?

Jenny: Not much of an impression was made on the first

meeting. Then I saw him again after I moved there. Five months later, he made me laugh hysterically, the hardest I'd laughed in a long time. I thought, "This guy's great." He happened to show up the next day in the building to see a friend, and I had this really bizarre experience, which is hard to describe, but it was like the room kind of *warbled*. I sensed this feeling in my body like this person is going to be in my life for a very long time. I don't know how, I don't know what capacity, but he is.

JJ: I've actually had the same experience, as well. How did your body feel?

Jenny: It wasn't a chemical reaction that says, "I'm really hot for that guy." It wasn't that at all; it was very interesting. My heart felt ease and calm, no rush, no hastiness. *I'm not sure who you are, but you're going to be in my life for a long time.*

JJ: How old were you and what was the state of the way you were taking care of yourself at that time?

Jenny: I was 27, and my fitness and health were better than they had ever been.

JJ: Truly?

Jenny: Truly, yes. At that point, I was still exercising. I would say that I was pretty darn compulsive about my exercise. I was doing 2 to 2 ½ hours of exercise a day because I was teaching dance, but my eating was the healthiest it had been at that point. Up until that point, for me, a good week would be binging two to three nights a week—that was a good week. At this point, it was one night every couple of weeks. I was having a lot of fun. I was doing work that I loved. My life was becoming more my own than it had ever been. I was following my intuition more than I had ever.

JJ: Would you say that you were happy independently, meaning you didn't need anyone in your life to make you happy?

Jenny: Absolutely. You know at that age, I was dating three guys, and I'm not a dater of multiple people. It was just easy, and I was having fun. My work was really engaging. I felt strong and enthusiastic. Now I'm 41, so I look back and can see there was still an undercurrent of panic with regards to my body. It was so much less than it had been. It used to rule my social life, and it didn't at that time.

JJ: And when it ruled your social life, what kind of relationships did you have?

Jenny: I didn't have any. No, I mean I had relationships with friends, girlfriends. I had a boyfriend who was so melancholy; he was just a mirror of me. He was an artist and very romantic and had a very hard time making a living, a very hard time taking care of the external business of his life. So I had relationships; they just weren't sustainable.

JJ: Can you make a connection between how you were treating yourself and the kind of relationships you had?

Jenny: Oh, completely. Oh, my God, yes. When I attracted Aaron, I was so much stronger. He's a strong, get-it-done, disciplined-focused individual. That is where I was. I was in a place of taking charge of my life. Of course, I attracted somebody who really knew how to take charge of his life. He was also very kind. You know, that piece had never been a problem for me. I was a sensitive, tenderhearted person. I think a lot of my eating was about squashing all the emotion and all the feelings because I was always putting everybody else first. I can absolutely make a connection. No question about it.

JJ: So you had found your husband and were the healthiest you had been since you were 12. What happened next?

Jenny: I got married, and we were both working. I really wanted to have a child. I got pregnant really easily, and it was wonderful. I had felt wave of panic about this body of mine, could it be trusted? I went into therapy and worked with a woman who specialized on body trauma. What I came to understand in that process was that it was no longer about me. I was bringing another life into this world; and so, I took impeccable care of myself. The really disciplined teacher in me took over, and I was really conscious. *I'm tired; I'm going to sleep. I'm hungry; I'm going to eat. I am going to eat foods that are nourishing for this child.* Because of that, I had a fantastic pregnancy.

The irony of all ironies is that it was the best I've ever felt in my life. The sense of really appreciating, listening, and taking care of my body was really exciting. The reward was that my body, after my first child, was truly the best body I've ever had. There was no baby weight. I had lost weight after the birth of my child, and he was eight pounds and four ounces. I looked at myself in the mirror and said, "How did this happen?" I was super fit.

JJ: It came from a place of love.

Jenny: It was complete, total, non-negotiable respect for my body and this life. After he was born, I had the opposite of post-partum. I had like post-partum bliss. I felt so powerful and strong. I was on fire about giving birth to this child. I had a home birth, and it was *wow!* Women are amazing! It was like an awakening to women because we are amazing.

After that, I started studying dance therapy and opened my own practice. I started a business. That went on for the next five years, and then I got pregnant with my daughter. I had a healthy pregnancy, but was a little bit more stressed because of already having a child and a business to manage. When she was born, she had digestive issues. She was allergic to 13 things, was covered in a rash, and it was extraordinarily stressful. I had to sell my practice, and I got pretty depressed. Looking back on that, I was at a place in my life where I had done so much inner work and outer work that I thought there has got to be some bigger reason for this happening. I was pulled in so many directions with what to do to get her better. The one thing I wouldn't do is just relax with her. Something I'd never been able to do is just slow down and chill out.

My daughter was really unhappy most of the time, and of course, I was exhausted. She wouldn't sleep well. She wouldn't nurse well. It was just a train wreck. One of her preschool teachers just scooped her up one day and got her to get quiet and fall asleep. I really liked this teacher. She was relaxed and happy, just like one of these women who looks like she thinks, "I'm just happy with who I am." This teacher got her to fall asleep. She looked at me and she said, "You just need to let go. Stop trying so hard to fix her and stop making her wrong. Stop focusing on her illness and start focusing on her health. Just try it. Only pay attention to what is perfect, what is healthy and try it." My daughter fell asleep in her arms, and I started crying. I was tired, stressed, and sad that my daughter was always uncomfortable and had this rash. "Okay, would you try it?" she asked, "Yeah, I'll do it."

In that month, I realized that I needed to stop nursing. *Maybe I'm part of the problem?* I stopped nursing her and overnight she started healing. She slept the longest she'd ever slept in over a year. The next morning, she started clearing up. My breast milk was making my daughter sick. I realized that I needed to listen and follow this little baby. She started to get better; now she's six and fabulous, wonderful, healthy, and vibrant. It was a slow progression of me slowing down, relaxing for the first time in my life, and coming full circle. I said, "The buck's going to stop here. You're not going to inherit all this food pathology and body pathology. We're going to walk through this world and know that you're perfect just the way you are. And, I'm perfect just the way I am." That is really what got me to today. I attracted incredible people in my life and you are a part of that team, JJ. When I started doing the *6 Week Beach Body Program*, I was coming out of that slow down period. I had really put my attention on listening to what my children's needs were.

JJ: What was going on with your life when you called me?

JT: My husband was getting his Ph.D., and I decided it was time to turn back to me. I was in transition. We had just moved to a new state. I didn't know anybody, and it was a totally new environment. My children were both entering school, so that was like a new phase of motherhood. I was ready to get back to the place of "what do I need now?"

JJ: What did you need?

JT: I signed up for your program because I knew I needed support in my whole health. It wasn't typical for me to reach out for support. This time, I knew I needed professional support, and I didn't want somebody that was mono-focused. I needed a broader perspective. When I found out about your program, I thought, "This is it! This is what I need. I need this balanced and upbeat approach. I need the science and the nutrition."

I wanted to lose weight and feel my vitality. I wanted to feel healthy again. I wanted to feel like Jenny, separate from being a mom or spouse again, but Jenny in a new calm, grounded way. Not running constantly, over functioning, and overextending myself, which is how I spent most of my life. *I don't want to do this alone.*

I know I won't be able to do it alone. I need support. I want to really trust the people I'm going to lean on. I had always been trying diets and none of them ever worked for long. I had done Weight Watchers, Nutri-System, The Zone Diet, the Atkins Diet, and Raw Foods Diet. This was the first time since college that I had said, "Okay, let's sign up for a program and get support."

JJ: Do you know why you wanted to lose weight? Was it to gain control?

Jenny: Absolutely. Yes. That pretty much sums it up.

JJ: You were at the place of feeling out of control. Feeling like your life wasn't yours?

Jenny: That's absolutely right. Even after all that I've done, my life still is not in my control. I felt like I was carrying around this extra weight. I didn't feel in control. It's true. That's it.

JJ: Let's take it a step further. You wanted to feel like you were in control. But then the next step is, "I want to feel control so I can feel . . ." Fill in the blank.

Jenny: I want to feel in control so that I can feel truly free in any situation and come and go as I please.

JJ: Part of it is control. Part of it is freedom. What's in freedom? Is freedom also a sense of acceptance and love? Most people can relate to feeling out of control. Feeling like there's extra weight on them, whether it is 5 pounds, 50 pounds, or 150 pounds. Whatever the number is, people can relate to feeling out of control and wanting to get the weight off. You started our program because you knew it wasn't just about the weight. You had taken off the weight before in all these other programs that you had done, right?

Jenny: Oh, yeah, but I gained it back immediately. I wasn't digging deep enough. I wasn't mining out the muck; I wasn't going to the root of it. It's true.

JJ: Did you have any ah-ha moments during the *6 Week Beach Body Program* that was different than the diets you've done before?

Jenny: Wow, yes. The first words that come to me are the sense of less is more. I really learned about the efficiency of exercise, realizing that after all the time that I've spent teaching movement that I wasn't being efficient in my workout; I could really get a huge benefit from being more efficient. Learning to exercise safely was a huge piece. Realizing I wasn't getting nearly enough protein. When I started actually eating enough protein, I started feeling calmer, more grounded, and stopped craving sugar. That was huge. Realizing that the master cleanse I had done in the past was not a good idea for me. I learned that a detoxification should be something that's non-damaging. I had done a cleanse before and really lost muscle mass and had damaged my body. Doing a good detox taught me that shouldn't happen. Something that was said that really stuck out was that being focused on what's wrong with your body is actually a very selfish state of being. It keeps you constantly circumventing what's not right and always having to solve problems; it keeps you over-focused on yourself. Actually accepting yourself and appreciating yourself is a less selfish thing to do. I had never heard it put in those words, and that was really helpful.

JJ: What happened when you did the body image exercises?

Jenny: Oh, it was pretty emotional. I had an experience of what I was giving my daughter in appreciating myself. Discovering that just the act of me appreciating myself and accepting myself just as I am, no matter what, was setting a good example, and it was my responsibility as a mother. It was the first time I had experienced this sense of responsibility around self-acceptance. This is not an indulgence. This is a responsibility that I have as a mother and as a woman to reverse this trend.

JJ: Afterwards, did you notice any difference with your relationship with your husband or your children?

Jenny: Ahhh, yes. Absolutely. First of all, as a result of doing the program, I manifested this scholarship to The Institute of Integrative Nutrition. That really came right at the end of doing the *6 Week Beach Body Program*. That was wonderful. It just dovetailed onto what I got in the program, which was bringing balance into my whole family. You know, I am the center of the house in my family. If mama's happy, everybody's happy. Period. If mama's balanced, everybody rides that wave—everybody.

The biggest piece that's come out of the program is owning up to my life when it is not balanced. *I need a little more protein. I need to do a detox. I need to say something. I need to listen to hypnotherapy. I need to do a body image exercise in front of the mirror. I need to drink some water. I need to get outside and change up my workout.* When I'm good, everybody else is good. So, that's the long answer for basically the change in my relationship. My husband is now saying, "Could you make a bunch of greens?" I give him a big liter bottle of water and say, "Drink this," and he does. There is so much more readiness and willingness to be healthy than there has been, bar none.

JJ: So your husband is more attentive?

Jenny: He is more attentive. All of a sudden he's really recognizing the work that I do. I believe that's because I'm taking better care of myself. There's more room for him to relax with all that I'm doing. So in general, life is pretty good.

JJ: Would you say life is the best it's been?

Jenny: Life is the most balanced it's been, absolutely. I am absolutely the strongest and the most at peace that I have ever been. No question. I have a sense of peace and balance that I've never had. The proof for me is that I'm continuously attracting clients while I'm in transition. We moved this year and started new schools for my kids. We have a new house and are going to new places. We don't know anybody, and I'm still attracting clients. My business is growing in spite of this, and I'm not overextending myself. That says a lot.

JJ: What advice would you give to someone who is where you were, struggling with an eating disorder or food addiction, maybe single or married and having these big issues with their body image? They have feelings about being out of control and focusing so much on the weight, what would you tell them?

Jenny: I would tell them every relationship that you have outside of you is a reflection of a part of yourself. If your perspective of the world is that your lovability is based on the pants size that you wear or whether you can fit into the right bathing suit in the exact way, then it's time to change your perspective. If you don't like the picture that you're projecting into the world, change your perspective. The worst that is going to happen is you're going to find out that you were wrong and that you are loveable just the way you are. Food is meant to be enjoyable and pleasurable, and so is exercise, and so is life.

JJ: What are three or four tools that had helped you get from the place you were to the place you are now?

Jenny: The first thing is to question your thoughts, not your sensations. Question your thoughts about who you are. Slow down; slow everything down. Listen to your heart and dare to follow your desires. Dare to follow your desires and celebrate that. Lastly, practice gratitude every day. Be diligent about beginning and ending your day with gratitude.

JJ: A lot of women think that they have to work out really hard to attract the right partner, wear the right clothes, or have the designer handbag. Did you do that to get your husband?

Jenny: No, he could care less about that. I mean, he appreciated it, and he regularly tells me now that he thinks I look great. I certainly don't look now like I did when we got together. My body has aged and has birthed two children. Everything has drooped. On my first date with my husband, when we walked by a window and there was a voluptuous bodice of a woman, like a baroque, and he said, "That's what a real woman looks like." She had curves and wasn't perfect.

JJ: Did you ever ask him what attracted him to you?

Jenny: He said, "You were just bright and fun, and you had a great sense of humor." He loved my laugh. I was doing something goofy when he first met me, I don't remember what it was. I'm sure he thought I was cute, but he said that I was the first woman he'd ever been with that didn't bore him. That's why he wanted to be with me.

JJ: Well, that's a great compliment. Even though you've been through a lot, I think you're journey has been about returning to a deep sense of self-respect. You had it when you were younger, but because your parents couldn't handle it, you acted differently in order to please them, get their approval, and their love. It was always in you; you just had to go back and find it. This journey was about returning back to you.

Jenny: It's in all of us. We all have to do our journey back to ourselves, the way we have to do it. If a woman really wants to have a partnership, she has to partner with herself first. She has to be that person she wants to be with for the rest of her life. Be the person you wish to see in your life, and they'll show up.

JJ: Thanks, Jen, for all your words of wisdom.

Jenny: You are very welcome. This is an exciting project.

Steps Jen Used to Attract the Love of Her Life— Herself

Step 1: Clean the Slate. Jen joined our *6 Week Beach Body Program* and did a body detox, as well as an emotional clean up around her self-image. She had some huge transformations during the body image section that healed some of the wounds from the past.

Step 3: A Food Love Affair. By adding more protein to her diet, Jenny could curb her cravings more easily. By working on the emotional connection with food through the *6 Week Beach Body Program*, Jenny was able to easily control portions and indulge in chocolate once a week. Her relationship with food was transformed in six weeks.

Step 5: Thank Your Lucky Stars: As she recommends to others, Jennifer Torok has practiced gratitude every day since becoming pregnant with her first child. Shifting the focus to what *is* working, rather than what is not, helped her heal her daughter.

Jennifer's journey, while unique to her, is common among many women. With the emphasis on body image, we judge ourselves from the outside in, instead of from the inside out. I interviewed Jen's husband, Aaron, to get an idea if men can see on the outside what women struggle with on the inside.

JJ: Hi, Aaron, thank you for your time. It occurred to me as I was speaking with Jenny that it would be really interesting and important for the readers to also hear your point of view. I just wanted to ask you some questions. Tell me what it was about Jenny that you were attracted to. Tell me about that first meeting.

Aaron: We're sort of opposite when it comes to professions. I'm more in technical disciplines, like engineering and physics. We met through a mutual friend, and I ended up moving into the same building where she lived. I met her at a party, and the first time was just kind of a nothing to speak of. We ended up seeing each other at another party a few months later during the holiday season and really hit it off that night. Then we ended up having this marathon first date. We spent the whole day together, and the rest is history.

JJ: Did you know early on that you were going to ask her to marry you?

Aaron: Yeah. I think so. I just had this notion that with her, I was never going to be bored. Most of the women that I met, even if I was attracted to them, were not that interesting. She really held my attention.

JJ: What other qualities did she have? Were you looking for a wife?

Aaron: No, not at all. I was definitely not on the hunt for a wife. I definitely wanted to be in a relationship, but I wasn't thinking about getting married.

JJ: You found the right person, so you couldn't deny it.

Aaron: I remember thinking that if I didn't ask her to marry me, I could end up regretting it for the rest of my life. I thought, "I'm going out and getting a ring to propose to her."

JJ: And how long had you been dating by that point?

Aaron: I think about four months.

JJ: Wow, that's pretty quick.

Aaron: Quick. Yeah. We were engaged for one year after that.

JJ: Good man. You figured it out and you said, "I'm not
          waiting any longer," and you caught her. At the time, did
          you know that she was having issues with her body and
          her self-image?

Aaron: Not really. Even after a while, I didn't really understand.
          I guess I just wasn't really aware of all of those issues in
          that way. I never really heard anybody talk about eating
          disorders or anything of that nature. I didn't understand
          that it was that deep for her; it was always on her mind
          and something that she was struggling with.

JJ: During the *6 Week Beach Body Program*, she had great
          experiences and kept a daily journal throughout the
          program. Did you see any change?

Aaron: Yeah. More than anything, it seems to me that she's been
          able to manage her anger and emotions better; she does
          not get so wrapped up in them like she used to. I've seen
          a difference in what she eats, as well.

JJ: Does she seem to be kinder to herself?

Aaron: She seems to be making better decisions for herself
          in terms of who she seems to be surrounding herself
          with. She recognizes earlier if someone else's energy is
          draining for her. She seems like she's able to navigate
          that better than before, where I think she's always tried
          to be very accommodating to everyone and try to please
          other people.

JJ: Great. Tell us about who Jenny is and her qualities? How
          would you describe her to someone who doesn't know

her?

Aaron: She is someone who deep down really wants to save the world. Jenny has very high ideals and tries to stick to those. At times, it makes it difficult, but in the end, she feels that's the only way to go. In this phase of her life, she's actualizing those ideas into her career. She's one of the most generous people that I've ever met. One of her best qualities is that she really takes a genuine interest in other people. She's extremely good at meeting people and connecting with them. She has that ability to really listen.

JJ: What three things would you tell single women who are looking for a relationship or who want to improve their relationship?

Aaron: People who are exercising and have healthy habits are going to feel better about themselves and more attractive. I notice that for myself, and I'm a man. Make sure you're doing something for yourself that makes you feel attractive, whatever that is. Have passion for something and be authentic.

JJ: That's some great advice. To recap: do something that makes you feel attractive, feel good about yourself, have a passion, and be authentic.

Aaron: Yes.

JJ: Thank you so much, Aaron.

Aaron: You're welcome.

Speaking with Aaron lets us see the blueprint Jennifer had created for him. A great teacher of mine once said, "The people who can really see you, see you already. The one's that do not see you, will not see you. You do not need to try, it will just be." Create who you are based on what you want to be and allow the right person who sees you, to find you.

Chapter 11

Midlife Perspective Change

"To love yourself right now, just as you are, is to give yourself heaven. Don't wait until you die. If you wait, you die now. If you love, you live now." Alan Cohen

Mike Burrichter has 25 years in the real estate industry, including acquisitions, asset management, leasing, property valuations, structuring participating loans, and joint venture transactions. Prior to joining the Strategic Partners team, Mike was Senior Acquisition Director with CBRE Investors, where he was one of the company's top investment professionals. CB Richard Ellis (CBRE) is the world's premier, full-service real estate services company. Operating globally, the firm holds a leadership position in virtually all of the world's key business centers. I started working with Mike in 2007 on creating a workout program that would get him results and fit his lifestyle.

JJ: When we met, you were single and starting to take better care of your body. Less than a year later, you manifested someone who also takes good care of her body and overall health. Your story is a perfect example of what *Fit 2 Love* is all about. Women can benefit from your point of view about the things that are important to men who are looking for a partner, wife, or mate. There is also a difference between guys who take care of their bodies for longevity and health versus men that are focused purely on esthetics, and you've lived it.

Where shall we start?

Mike: I'm 50 years old. I am an investor with a company of real estate funds based in downtown Los Angeles. I travel a lot for work. For example, next week, I'll leave Tuesday morning at 6:00 am and get back Friday night at 7:45 pm, and I will have gone to Chicago, Washington DC, Northern Virginia, and Tampa during the week. In order to take care of myself, it requires effort. I can't say I am disciplined, because that's never really been me. So, it is an effort to eat the right foods and get in quality exercise.

JJ: Have you always been active?

Mike: In high school, I participated in sports and intramurals and also played softball right after college. When I was younger, I didn't have to have a regimen. After that, I just gradually got pretty out of shape and then decided in my 30's to start working out. As I got into my early 40's, I realized that I needed some help with the workout. I also needed help with things like nutrition, and so while I would not describe myself as overly active, by virtue of my being single for 50 years, I've not been sedentary.

JJ: On a scale of 1 to 10, 1 being a couch potato, 10 being a professional athlete, where are you?

Mike: I'd probably be in the 5 to 7 range.

JJ: Originally, what motivated you to get started and take care of your health? Was there anything that triggered your commitment?

Mike: I went to the doctor for a checkup, and everything was fine except for my testosterone. It dawned on me that I could keep my weight under control and not be healthy. So, I had to really start looking at things like nutrition and sleep and dealing with stress and exercise, all in one bucket. For me, the idea was that I want to retire someday and still be active. A big part of it for me was dealing with my parents and their health issues, especially my mother. She has Parkinson's disease. It's pretty advanced, and she's only 72 now. She got it when she was around 50 years old. It effectively changed her whole life, and she has not been able to enjoy her later years. I thought to myself, *I don't want that.* I know there's no way I can prevent Parkinson's, but I can avoid so many other health issues by taking care of myself. A real quality set of senior years is possible. So then, when I got the tests back, I thought, I've really have to start taking this stuff seriously because I want to be able to do things. I'm killing myself at work. If I can't do anything when I finish working, what is it all for?

JJ: Absolutely. Your insight is something everyone needs. Unfortunately, for a lot of people, it takes situations like this to consider the future of their health. I'm so sorry to hear about your mother. No wonder you were taking care of yourself from a place of health, instead of just for aesthetics.

When we met, you were obviously in self-care mode. You had just signed up to do all kinds of health work, and then you signed up for my *90-Day Health and Body Makeover Program.* You were full-on committed to helping yourself lose weight and feel better. We worked on strengthening your muscles for hip stability and to reduce body fat. You lost some weight, and the pain in your hip was less than it had been in years, so we were meeting your goals?

Mike: Yeah. I did really well, until I started dating Polina and then living with her. Then it's been a lot harder. You warned me about that before I met her, and I didn't really understand what you were saying at the time. And now, I get it.

JJ: Yes, because new relationships always challenge our

self-care habits and time management.

Mike: Polina is as skinny as a rail and has the ability to keep candy all over the place. She's the type of person who can take the candy out the wrapper, take one bite, and then put the wrapper back on the shelf. When I see candy, I inhale it. Plus, I really haven't gotten into a full-on workout schedule since my hip surgery. It took almost four months until I could go to the gym. And then I had to really ease into it. Now I'm starting to go at it full tilt.

JJ: Part of this project is about women loving themselves and attracting a relationship based on self-love first. Usually a man can recognize that, yes? Can you tell the difference between women who don't like themselves and women who do?

Mike: Yeah. I mean, it's basically comparing a happy woman to an unhappy woman. It's the same for men. I think women stress a hell of a lot more about how they look than men do. Although, I know some men that come close to most women.

JJ: There's a healthy way and an unhealthy way to approach all of this, for example, from a place of fear or from love and respect. It's rewarding to work with clients and help them find ways to support themselves through loving and respecting their bodies, such as taking it seriously, giving it time, attention, effort, and maintaining the integrity of their body for the long haul. Instead of boot camps and crash diets that can make people lose weight really fast, but don't take into account the impact on the body, like wearing down the knee joints quickly, or what it can do to the liver in the long run. Part of it is instant gratification without understanding the consequences.

Mike: True. That's always been part of it for me, but when I met you, it was all about preparing myself for my senior years. The bottom line is it's not just about looking good and feeling good. I want to be able to do just about everything I could do when I was 20 years old. That's really enjoying life. No one wants to say, "*I can't do this anymore because I'm just too old or just too out of shape.*" I want to be able to enjoy physical activity. It's always going to be part of my life.

JJ: When we started working together, were you actively looking for a partner?

Mike: Yes, I was. I was single, and I have never been married. I found Polina after I started working with you, and we are living together now.

JJ: Were you clear about what you were looking for in a partner?

Mike: No. Just somebody that was nice. Somebody I was attracted to and not just physically, but overall. I had no criteria that I was aware of. I didn't want the "5'10" blonde" sort of thing.

JJ: So, looks were not that important to you?

Mike: Right.

JJ: Were there any other qualities that maybe you didn't define back then, but looking back now that you would have requested?

Mike: I don't know how to describe it. The two women I dated before ended up being more about the chemical thing, all about looks, and they ended up being pretty bad people. I just wanted somebody who was happy and not malicious. I wanted someone who is kind, warm, and doesn't take herself too seriously, over someone who is just hot. I wanted to be with someone who was open to living abroad and who had a healthy outlook, both physically and mentally.

JJ: What can you say about Polina and your relationship?

Mike: She's pretty easy going. We have mutual respect for each other. What makes this relationship different is that we workout together, and I like that.

JJ: Great! What is it about her personality, values, and behaviors that you respect? What do you admire most?

Mike: I'm not religious at all, but Polina is very spiritual. She studies with a healer, and she's really into self-help books. She keeps a notebook, and she writes things down all the time. Things like *I want to be nice today.* I really admire her for doing everything she can to be a good person. She's also pretty and takes care of herself. I have a ton of respect for someone who can figure out how to eat three meals a day, eat what they like, and never be hungry or have a weight problem. I've always had that problem. I'm about to go into a cocktail reception. There'll be finger food there, and I can overdo it so easily. I have never seen her do that.

JJ: One of my programs deals with this. Part of the *6 Week Beach Body Program* is about reprogramming the mind. It sounds like Polina has been programmed to think thin.

Mike: Yes. That's for sure.

JJ: It's a mindset, not a discipline. She probably doesn't struggle with it, right?

Mike: She doesn't. It looks like it's so easy for her, and it is so hard for me.

JJ: Well, I'm sure at one time in your life, you probably could eat whatever you wanted, and it didn't matter, correct?

Mike: Yeah. Pretty much.

JJ: The reality of aging is that the chemistry in the body
changes.

Mike: Yep. What is this program that you have?

JJ: The *6 Week Beach Body Program.* It is a set of hypnosis
               and creative visualization audios to listen to reprogram
               your mind. Eighty-eight percent of your mind is actually
               subconscious, so we're not aware of the feelings or
               the thoughts that we're having. When people deal
               with food issues and having lack of motivation with
               exercise, they usually think it's about willpower. It's not
               just about willpower. Some people, like Polina, do not
               struggle because it's part of their mindset. It's part of
               her relationship with food, her body, and exercise. It's
               ingrained in her, so it is not a struggle. On the flip side,
               some people are programmed the opposite way, so
               they think if they don't eat pasta, that they're missing
               something important in life. Or they may think that
               exercise is cruel and unnecessary, while others actually
               see exercise as stress relief and a critical part of their
               day. It depends on the mindset and the emotions that
               got attached to the thoughts. One of the fastest ways to
               change the subconscious mind is with hypnosis. Plus,
               there is nothing to do except listen to it.

Mike: I'll have to check it out.

JJ: Yes, you do. What advice can you give to single women
               who are looking for a man? What would you tell them to
               focus on?

Mike: First, does the guy have any values? Can you trust him?
               Does he have meaningful relationships with friends
               and family? Does he have a healthy mental and physical
               lifestyle? These are the questions I would recommend a
               woman use to evaluate the quality of a man.

JJ: Great, the emphasis is on the *woman* evaluating the man, instead of wondering if and how she will pass his evaluation. That's very empowering for a woman. Thanks, Mike. I appreciate your time with all of this.

Mike: You are very welcome. Glad I could help. I hope it makes a difference.

JJ: I am sure it will!

Steps Mike Used to Attract the Love of His Life

Step 1: Clean the Slate. While Mike did not do a formal detox, he embarked upon a serious change in how he approached his health. He started working with a doctor to regulate his hormones and increase his testosterone production back to a healthy level, he made adjustments to his diet, and he hired me for a three-month weight loss and exercise program.

Step 2: Sexual Fitness. Mike had a degenerative hip that was painful for many years. I built Mike an exercise program he could do while traveling to lose weight and strengthen his hip—he lost seven pounds in the first month and his hip pain reduced dramatically. He was also doing Pilates once a week for his hip and core. Mike felt good about the weight loss and was virtually pain free for months. When you focus on feeling good, you attract others who feel good, as well.

Step 5: Thank Your Lucky Stars: When Mike realized that he had control over the future health of his body in his senior years, he took immediate action investing in the longevity of his body. Looking around at how other people struggle can be the trigger to be thankful for what you have and wanting to work hard to keep it.

Mike's hip might have been a blessing in disguise to give him a warning of what could happen to his body as he aged. Changing the way he took care of his health changed the kind of person he attracted into his life. You do not have to have an injury or disease to shift your perspective about your future. I encourage you to get clear on what you do want, how you want your life to be, and then be grateful for what you have now.

Chapter 12

Superficial To Successful

"Unless your heart, your soul, and your whole being are behind every decision you make, the words from your mouth will be empty, and each action will be meaningless. Truth and confidence are the roots of happiness." **Anonymous**

Alexis Neely has built two different one million dollar businesses, published a bestselling book, and appeared on many of the top television shows as a legal expert, all while raising two kids and diving into the path of awakening. Today, she is an evolutionary strategist consulting with evolving entrepreneurs on how to build sustainable and make-a-difference businesses based on who they are and how they want to serve. Her groundbreaking Money Map technology and her LIFT Foundation System make this possible. Follow Alexis on Twitter at www.twitter.com/AlexisNeely and get on her list for an advance copy of her eBook, *Your Soul's Evolution Through Life and Business: 3 Keys to Waking Up and Integrating Your Great Work.* www.AlexisMartinNeely.com

JJ: Tell us a little bit about yourself.

Alexis: I help entrepreneurs build business models and structures around their greatest gifts; I've been in business for myself since 2003. The biggest challenge I face throughout my adult life has been my relationships because I was always attracting people who saw me as somebody who

would take care of them more than myself. I put other
people and their emotional and physical needs before
my own. That meant that I attracted men, like my first
husband, who ultimately became dependent upon me.
They really didn't share the same vibrations that I had
and that I really wanted in my life. As a result, there was a
tendency for conflict. I would feel resentful, and I wouldn't
communicate what it was that I wanted or needed because
I was occupied with second-guessing myself about what I
deserved, what was right, and what could I ask for.

JJ: When you got married the first time, what was your self-
          care regimen? How did you take care of yourself?

Alexis: I didn't take care of myself at all. It was really quite
          interesting because back in 2001-2002, I was working at a
          big law firm. I was really unhappy there, so I hired a coach
          to help me. All of a sudden, she started talking to me about
          self-care, "When's the last time you went to the dentist?
          When's the last time that you exercised? When's the last
          time you got your hair cut or a pedicure?"

          I was really quite pissed off because here I was paying her
          to coach me about my business, and she was asking me all
          these questions. "Why are you asking me these questions?
          I want you to help me figure out why I'm so unhappy in my
          work."

          She said, "Well, it has to start with you taking care of
          yourself, because if you don't take care of yourself, you're
          never going to be happy in anything that you do." That was
          a big wake-up call for me because I had never taken care
          of myself. I never spent money on myself. With a baby at
          home, taking the time to go work out or spending money
          on a pedicure, even a haircut was not going to happen. All
          my free time and money went to my family. What she really
          helped me to realize was that if I didn't take care of myself
          for my family, I would not be happy in my business at all.

JJ: Did you at that point change your life and start exercising and taking better care of yourself?

Alexis: I did. That was the first time. It actually saved my life, in a kind of random way. I started to drive into the office about an hour early to work out downtown, instead of sleeping in and sitting in rush hour traffic; it seemed like a good plan. One morning, I was driving on the freeway, and the sun was coming up over the freeway. All of a sudden, the car right in front of me swerved. As it swerved, I realized there was this huge roll of carpet in the middle of the freeway in front of me. I had two choices. I could either hit the roll of carpet or try to swerve and go around it. I'm in this little Volkswagen GTI, so I decided to swerve. As I spin the wheel to the right very fast, all of a sudden, I'm spinning across the highway. I hear this voice in my head; it says, "turn into the spin, turn into the spin." I start turning my wheel, and I come to a screeching halt, facing the wrong way on the highway up against the fence. I get out of the car, and I'm shaking. I look around, and there was no damage. Well, a little scratching on the side of my car. All of a sudden, I hear another voice that says, "Get it the car and move, move, now!" So I get in the car and literally seconds later, exactly where I was standing, another car comes spinning and slams head first into the median exactly where I'd been standing. It was the voice in my head that really saved my life. I had never had voices in my head before that told me anything helpful. Until that point, all the voices in my head would say things to me like, "What's wrong with you? Why can't you fit in? You're not good enough?" It was a constant barrage of negativity.

When I started exercising self-care, it opened up another voice inside of me—a voice that I think was trying to talk to me all along, but because I had always ignored it, it was like a child that doesn't get enough attention. It starts to exhibit negative behaviors. And, that's when it happened for me. I'd ignored myself for so long that my interior voice had started to funnel negative patterns of talking that disappeared when I started taking care of myself. That was the first period in my life that I really started taking care of myself. It had a huge impact on my life.

I didn't always keep taking care of myself after that. My life has always been reflective of the amount of self-care that I've been giving myself at various points. When I started taking care of myself for the first time ever, it led me to start my own business and leave the big law firm. Practicing self-care helped me to realize that I wasn't ever going to be happy working for someone else, and I gained the confidence to start my own business.

JJ: Where were you with exercise and your relationships right before I met you several years ago?

Alexis: When I started my own business, I was extremely busy, and I stopped taking care of myself because I got caught up in the "I don't have enough time" syndrome. It was right after my divorce, which came out of this renewed commitment to start taking care of myself. I'd been in my business for maybe a year and a half. I was still holding all of the baby weight from my two year old. I'd gained quite a bit with each of my kids.

This one Sunday, I was sitting on the couch and feeling like a total slug: lethargic, unmotivated, and really unhappy. I said to myself that day, "Okay, Alexis. You've got to do something because this is not working." I made a commitment to myself the next day to go to yoga. In that yoga class, something opened up in my body. Before that time, I had resigned myself to never having sex again. I was 28 years old and married, I had a business and kids, and I was not attracted to my husband. I decided I'd never have sex again. *It's fine. Oh, well. I've got the business, I've got the kids, and I'm married. It's all good.* If you ever find yourself saying that, it's not good. It's not all good. It's not okay.

JJ: You are a very attractive woman, so it's interesting to hear
           you say that because I would assume that a lot of women
           who are currently in sexless marriages or sexless lives
           would look at you and say, "She'd never say that!"

Alexis: But I did. The way my body looked and felt reflected that.
           I was probably still attractive back then, but I didn't feel
           attractive. I felt terrible. I felt like a slug. I felt lethargic.
           I didn't feel good in my body. I was holding all this baby
           weight from my second child, working constantly, and not
           doing any sort of physical exercise at all. I just felt terrible.

           In the yoga class, something literally opened up inside of
           my body. All of a sudden, I reconnected with my body and
           recognized that I'd been living in this numbness for such a
           long time, and I couldn't do it anymore. Ultimately, that led
           me to recognize that I was lying to myself. My relationship
           wasn't going to get better, and I needed to start making
           big changes, which led to a divorce and to me beginning to
           really take care of myself in a different way. I appreciated
           myself differently.

JJ: After your divorce, you dated a few men and had long-
           term relationships with them. What was your relationship
           to your body, fitness, and health through each of those
           relationships?

Alexis: It was all about the way I looked. It wasn't about my health.

JJ: It was superficial, and, therefore, those relationships did
           not work out. Deep inside, your inner being fought the
           whole idea of exercise because it was only about how you
           looked, which is probably why it never clicked. Your higher
           self knew it should be about something deeper than that.

Alexis: Yeah. Through all of those relationships, I was more
           focused on the superficial. It started to shift when I began
           Tantra and work on my spiritual practice. When I was
           with Dave, my ex-boyfriend, I found that the basis of our
           relationship really became work and was not working

out. We just worked all the time. He got into an exercise regimen, but it was more about the physical appearance, rather than what I'm calling health at all levels. We had a good relationship in many ways, but it wasn't ultimately fulfilling because it wasn't multi-dimensional enough. It really was focused on working and making as much money as possible. Any sort of exercise or anything that we were doing at that point was on the ego level.

During that relationship, I started to gain weight again. You know what they say about getting fat and happy. I was happy. I remember trying on clothes because I was doing a lot of TV at that point, and I couldn't fit into any of them. When I began to exercise and take care of my body again, it still wasn't from a place of health at all levels. It was from a place of *I'm fat! I need to lose this weight. I need to be able to fit into my clothes again!*

Over the past year, so much had changed. One of the biggest shifts definitely has been on this deeper level of health— having a deeper level of awareness and commitment to what I am calling health at all levels. I am raising my vibration so I can hold a different level of energy. When that happens, I attract to me a different caliber of people. I made a commitment about a year ago to really only be in healthy relationships; whether it's a business relationship, personal relationship, or any kind of relationship, it must be with people who are really on a conscious path, who are vibrating at a higher energy level.

JJ: When you made that shift, did you change anything about your self-care?

Alexis: Yeah. When I made this decision, I really changed everything. First of all, I found the right form of exercise for me, which was really important. In the past, I tried to do other people's preferred form of exercise. High intensity exercise for 20 minutes is perfect for me. I learned how to eat smaller portions and really began to maintain this commitment to the truth of what is true for me and what is really right for me.

I let go of my entire team in my business: completely deconstructed my entire business. I ended my relationship with Dave, even though from the outside looking in, anybody would say that it was a great relationship. It was, but it wasn't the best ever relationship. Same thing with my business, it was a great business, but it wasn't the best ever business. I began to let go of the things that were good, but weren't excellent, in favor of really creating the aligned life that I wanted to have.

It was during that time that Russell came back into my life. He and I had been friends for quite a long time but did not have any romantic attraction. I was totally not interested in him romantically. We kept trying to coach each other because he's a relationship coach, and I'm a business coach, but it kept not working. It was really sticky and uncomfortable. Then he came back into my life, he asked me on a date, and all of a sudden, things opened up. It was interesting because I remember when we first started dating, I was really looking at him and recognizing *wow, this guy is everything on my list in terms of the way that he lives his life. He was living the kind of life I wanted to have: a health at all levels life.* This was what I wanted.

JJ: How quickly did you know that Russell was the person you were going to marry?

Alexis: We started dating on July 26th, and he asked me to marry him on September 1st. We got married on September 3rd. So it was very fast—very, very, very, *very* fast. I think what allowed it to be so fast is the fact that both of us are committed to something that is much greater than either one of us. We are really both committed to this idea of health at all levels, as opposed to, again, being part of this one-dimensional focus on the way that we look or the amount of money that we make. It's about this deeper commitment to doing our great work and really serving at a very deep level with a tremendous amount of self-care. In fact, one of the best things about him coming into my life is that he really, truly supports me. I get caught up in work, in business, and in my family, so then my self-care suffers. One of the things that is really great about him and that we argue about, which is nice, is the degree of self-care that I take for myself. He won't stand for me not to make self-care a priority, which is really refreshing. It's great.

JJ: That's awesome. For single women or women in a relationship that aren't happy and want something better, what advice would you give them?

Alexis: Focus on yourself. Focus on becoming the person that you would need to be to attract the person that you want to be with. Ask yourself, "Who and how would I need to be to attract this person that I really want to be with?" Then become that person: someone who is full of health.

I moved to Colorado about a year ago. One of the reasons I moved was because I found myself getting very caught up in the ego part of living in LA, with TV and all. One of the things I started doing when I moved here is running. You might remember, JJ, that I never liked to run before. But here, all of a sudden, I do. I have no idea why, but I do. So, I started running regularly. I climbed my first 14,000 foot mountain this summer. And, lo and behold, I've attracted someone who likes those things: who loves the outdoors and loves nature. Guess what? That was on my list. But how could I ever have attracted someone who loved to be in nature if I wasn't being in nature? Become the person you would want to be with.

JJ: What do you think are some of the biggest mistakes women make when looking for a relationship?

Alexis: Not holding out long enough, being so desperate for a relationship that we settle. I can use that word because

I've been that, too, so I can say that. We say yes to the first person that shows us attention, even if it's not the right person. That comes from low self-esteem. I had low self-esteem for a long time. I wasn't willing to hold out because I didn't want to be alone. I was very willing to turn a blind eye to things that I should have been willing to see and said no rather than saying yes so quickly. I think if we look at some of my relationships, we can certainly see that.

Be really clear about what it is that you want, and then don't settle for less. When you settle for less, you block the ability for the right person that has all the things you want in your life—so don't settle. Don't think that you need to get into a monogamous relationship so quickly, either. I see this as another place where a lot of women limit their options too soon. It's okay to date multiple people. You don't have to be in a committed, steady relationship right away.

The whole summer before I met Russell, I was dating for the first time. I was dating lots of different types of people and got to see lots of different types of energy. Therefore, when I met Russell, I could say to myself, *I've seen what's out there. I've really looked for what I'm looking for, and I see that we line up on so many levels.* That doesn't mean we line up on every single level, but what we are both committed to is growth as the continuous process of really looking at yourself and being willing to grow together.

JJ: Can you see how you created the blueprint from which someone else learns how to treat you? Fitness is a mirror to your level of self-care. If you are not willing to love and cherish yourself, why would you expect someone else to?

Alexis: That's absolutely right. You've got to love yourself first. It's absolutely, positively true. Sometimes that might mean letting go of the relationship that you do have and not being afraid that you're going to be alone forever. Is the relationship that you're in now serving you? If it's not, be willing to let it go in favor of something that does. What could you do to show the universe that you love yourself? When you show the universe that you really love yourself, then other people can start to love you back. This cultivates a level of energy that is magnetic for people when you start to take care of yourself on a very deep level with fitness, nutrition, the space that you live in, and the relationships that you allow to be in your life. And then, you can pick and choose who you're with. You don't have to settle.

JJ: Excellent. Your transformation is very inspiring for women. I know you have found the perfect partner, and I wish you a lifetime of health and happiness!

Alexis: Thanks, JJ. This is an exciting project.

JJ: Thank you, Alexis, so much!

Steps Alexis Used to Attract the Love of Her Life

Step 1: Clean the Slate. Alexis did a life detox: she moved, ended her relationship, and deconstructed her whole business team. She knew she wanted more out of each of these areas of her life, so she created the space for that to happen by cleaning the slate.

Step 2: Sexual Fitness. High intensity, short duration interval training is what Alexis has been committing to for over a year—it fits into her busy schedule easily. She added running when she moved and has made a commitment to finding a man who would allow her to stay in her feminine.

Step 3: A Food Love Affair. Alexis changed her diet by focusing more on fruits, vegetables, and fish. She wanted to eat food that would raise her vibration, so she cut out meat and processed foods.

Step 5: Thank Your Lucky Stars. As long as I have known her, Alexis makes the best of every situation and finds *the lesson* for her. While most people ask, "Why did this happen to me?" Alexis invites the lesson to help her grow to the next level. Having this outlook not only has made her a millionaire, it helped her attract the love of her life.

Use these tools in the best way that works for you. As Alexis pointed out, she found what worked best for her schedule so she could commit to exercise on a regular basis. Take action, trust that it will all work out, and enjoy your journey.

Chapter 13

A Man's Spiritual Journey

"Our ultimate freedom is the right and power to decide how anybody or anything outside ourselves will affect us."
Stephen R. Covey

Casey Capshaw began his professional career in Los Angeles working in a number of positions at Mark Burnett Productions on television shows such as Survivor, Apprentice, Contender, and many others. Realizing he wanted more out of life than television could offer, he now resides in Boulder, Colorado and is Director of Marketing for Inspire Commerce, a for-benefit merchant services and eCommerce upstart. He also volunteers with men's groups, men's transformational workshops, and relationship work. We met through Facebook, when a friend referred me to his amazing blog post about finding his love. I was so taken by his depth and willingness to share his honest, open heart.

JJ: Thanks, Casey, for sharing your story. At what point did it begin?

Casey: I have always seen life as a unique journey, an adventure. This has shown up in my life as travel, taking calculated risks, and always aiming to live a life less ordinary. At 19, I took my first trip east of the Mississippi on a solo backpacking trip to Ireland and the UK. At age 21, I traveled to Kenai, Alaska and signed up for the summer commercial salmon fishing. At 25, I ran the LA marathon on 2 months of training; and that same year, I spent 3 months backpacking through Costa Rica on about 12 bucks a day. I have quit jobs many people would kill to have and taken others most wouldn't do for any about of money always in search of the deeper truth for me. I am not very good at settling for less than what I really want. It is fair to say I enjoy exploring.

JJ: Wow! That's amazing. You are quite the traveler and have a low tolerance for anything except the exceptional in life. I practice living the same way as best I can. Your passion is not surprising because what stuck out in your blog post was the depth of your emotional adventure and your willingness to share it.

Casey: Personally, I have always asked the deeper questions about life. I see my life as an ever-unfolding evolutionary process. To that end, I dive in headfirst to philosophy, eastern spirituality, Integral theory, shamanism, personal development, therapy, bodywork, and any other tool or methodology I can find to increase my freedom and fullness in this world.

JJ: And because of this work, you are now in love?

Casey: Yes. I am in love. Humbly. Overwhelmingly. Completely.

JJ: Congratulations! In your blog, you outline the steps it took you to be the person you needed to be to attract your love. Let's talk about some of those. Step one was doing your own inner work.

Casey: I always thought that I just had not found the right person. Instead, I learned that I was not being the right person. I was not open to the love I thought I wanted in my life and not able to see it, even if it was right in front of me. My journey of opening to love required me to turn inward and do some work on myself. What I mean by *work* is the act of getting on a path toward wholeness by taking a look at the darker, subtler, shadow parts of myself that I had not been unable or unwilling to see. For me, this work started with meditation practice in Zen Buddhism. Zen meditation became foundational in my development and allowed me to stay present when feelings such as intensity and fear came up. I also studied a lot of Eastern, Western, and Integral philosophy giving me a solid framework to understand how the pieces of my self fit together as I uncovered the hidden ones.

The real work, the hard psychological stuff, started with a men's personal development workshop that cracked my heart wide open. I revealed a pattern or shadow that had been unconsciously running my life the whole time. I saw how I was subconsciously not opening my heart, not letting people really *in* for fear of being hurt.

With this realization, I dove in to self-discovery with both feet, hoping to uncover more of my *shadow* and discover more of who I really am. I created The New Man podcast with Tripp Lanier, and we talked to dozens of experts in the personal development field. I worked with a therapist, a somatic therapist (body and energy focused), life coaches, and attended relationship workshops.

Through this work, I uncovered the ways shadow was running my life. Paramount in these discoveries was the revelation of a deeper fear of not being good enough. I have learned that I never want to feel like I am not good enough, and that is a deep underlying emotion that is with me often, if not all the time. Part of my path to greater wholeness is the acceptance of *not good enough* and appreciation for the creative energy it can bring to my life. I continually put the insights I received in this work to practice in all the relationships in my life with mixed results, but I am always learning.

JJ: You are not alone in that. We are all always learning or at least given daily opportunities to do so. Not everyone is comfortable with looking in the mirror and owning some of these patterns, which is why it's important to share the work you have done with women, as well as men, to let people know that we all have fears and shadow sides to us. When it came to looking for a partner, did you know what you wanted?

Casey: I always had an image of love in my mind. I knew a few things I really felt were important to me in a relationship. I knew what I stood for as a man, but I really wasn't all that clear on what I wanted in a partner. I would just sort of go about my life and react to what showed up. I needed to get clear on what I wanted in a partner. I mean I got really clear. I am not sure where I picked up this exercise, but someone suggested I literally make a list of things I wanted in a partner. I did, and I got really specific. I am talking specific–down to hair color, what she smells like, how she handles conflict, and what parts of my life I wanted to share with her. From this place of clarity, I had options on what to include in my life, and what to let go of. I could see the things that were core values of mine, essential things I wanted to share in partnership. I got really clear on what the green lights and red lights would look like, and I started paying attention to that when I met new people. It wasn't like I was checking boxes off a checklist, but more an orienting to where my core values would line up in relationship.

JJ: A similar exercise, my treasured list of what I wanted in a man, helped me attract my husband. On our first date, he even asked what was on my list.

              Getting clear about what is wanted makes it possible to recognize when it is found. My list also served me by constantly redefining what I wanted. When I first started the list and would attract the qualities that I had asked for, I would soon discover that I might have made a mistake. These trial and error situations are what helped to form my final list. I'm grateful for the time it took to get it right!

Another suggestion for women looking for a relationship is to clean the slate and start fresh. Did you do anything to symbolize a new beginning? My husband took eight months to ask me out because he was preparing for me. What did you do?

Casey: Absolutely. I cleared the decks. I started to notice all the things in my life that were distracting me from the relationship I truly wanted. I got serious about making the real thing happen and started feeling the pain of being out of integrity with this. It was time to clear the decks.

I had heartfelt conversations with the women in my life that I had close connections with, but knew were not the relationships I was looking for. I needed to clear up the gray areas and make real space in my life for what I truly wanted. This was not easy. I had to face my integrity faults directly and clean them up. I sat with tears, both mine and theirs. My shadow triggers of *caretaker* and *not good enough* were pushed, but I could see them arise and not be driven by them. My heart was wide open, and I was clear in my intention. In the end, in each case there has been mutual appreciation, gratitude for the connection we shared, and open clarity about where the boundaries now stand. In my personal experience, this clearing made space for that real relationship to happen. The universe responded almost immediately. I met my love soon after.

JJ: What an amazing journey to clean up your past relationships. Creating space in your heart is as important as creating space in your home—actually, it may be more important. Moving stuff around to accommodate another's things is a heck of a lot easier than facing old hurts and wounds about what went on in past relationships. Your example of cleaning the slate would be the optimal wish for anyone carrying around old baggage in their minds and hearts that make them unable to open up to love. I admire your strength and willingness.

What can you share about your love?

Casey: I could write an entire book about what is amazing about this woman the way the love from her heart utterly shines through her ocean-blue eyes, the way she commands a room with a soft, yet powerful, grace, her ability to show up as a flowing radiant girl or a fierce, focused woman, depending on what the situation invites or demands.

The biggest thing I love about her, bigger than who she is, the things we have in common, or the shared goals we have for our lives, is her profound ability to work with me through whatever comes up in our relationship. She is resourced with her own support system that she relies on when challenges arise in her life. She shows up for me fully. If anything comes up in our relationship, for me or for her, she has a calm presence that seems to hold us while we work it out. This is such a gift for me. It allows me to drop that *caretaker* impulse and meet her on even ground. I trust her so deeply. In this *container*, our relationship has become totally open. We share what arises for us, as it arises, and ask for what we need. What a gift to be in a relationship like this.

JJ: For the women that are out there looking for a man, what else would you advise them to do that worked for you in attracting a partner?

Casey: Be open. I really identify with the old saying: *the older I get, the less I know.* Life is more complex and mysterious than I will ever comprehend. In my case, I opened to the mystery, to the reality that I had no idea where that special person would walk into my life. She could have been the barista at the coffee house near my office or the bohemian folk singer whose voice kept distracting me from my buddies' political conversation. I dropped my expectations and just opened up. I opened to everybody I could. It became an awareness practice for me and seemed to have a positive effect on everybody I encountered. I think that would work for men or for women.

JJ: Great advice for living life to the fullest, but especially if you want to attract more love into your life.

Casey: Yes! I also followed my heart. Sometimes I am drawn to things or people without knowing why in any conscious way. I notice that when I let myself follow this *heart wisdom*, I am usually led into amazing, rewarding, or at the very least, educational experiences. When I met the woman I came to love, I was following my heart. I took a risk, moved toward what I was drawn to and did not get into why. From this place, I was not really attached to any outcome, just curious and present. Our first encounter was easy, exciting, and deep. I trust that deep inner voice and am open to the mystery. I give myself permission to follow this force without knowing why.

JJ: Yes, that was true for me, as well. Even with a clear list, there were *red flags*, but I followed my heart. I knew everything would be fine. I am usually the analyst, but I definitely surrendered, followed my heart, and was open to possibility. Did you have a similar experience?

Casey: There are enough green lights in my current relationship that I am ready to go for it. I have no idea what this will look like, and I am loving it. I am throwing away the lists and doing my best to drop expectations. I want to be completely present to what is arising in the moment. Sure, a part of me is keeping an eye out for major red flags or deal breakers, but I keep my focus on what is there and what is working. If something is not quite working, I set the intention to work together to get closer to synergy in that area. The love in my heart is literally creating a *container* for the relationship: a safe place where anything can be explored and worked through. That is where I am right now. For me, this path has been incredibly rewarding, and I wouldn't have had it any other way. I am on to the next adventure, deep authentic and committed relationship, and look forward to the challenges and opportunities this next part of the journey will undoubtedly reveal.

JJ: Let's close with three things you'd tell women to concentrate on while getting ready to find their mate. What is important for women to know about what men are looking for?

Casey: Relationships are a terrible place to *get* something. If you are looking to get something from relationships, that is a great sign to stop, take a breath and look inside. There is huge opportunity for growth *before* you move to share yourself with another.

Fully explore your feminine side. Women are so much better than we are at inhabiting the feminine expression of humanity. Life calls women to also inhabit their masculine expression, which is important and beautiful, but don't forget about your essence. When a woman shows up deeply feminine for me, it calls forth my deep masculine, and the polarity is irresistible.

Play. What a beautiful game dating and courtship is. Enjoy the journey of exploration of yourself and the search for that compliment out there in the world.

JJ: Thanks, Casey, for this amazing advice. I wish you all the love your heart can hold and appreciate your willingness to share your story with the world.

Steps Casey Used to Attract the Love of His Life

Step 1: Clean the Slate. Casey's detoxification was emotional. He went back through his relationships and looked in the mirror to see the kind of person he was projecting to others. Coming to closure, as well as gaining insights from each past relationship, allowed him to release any old negative energy holding him back from creating space for a new love.

Step 2: Sexual Fitness. Casey got in touch with his true masculinity through his work in men's transformational groups and workshops to uncover shadow parts of himself that were sabotaging him from being open to love. Being with other men in this kind of work supports the integrity and honor of being a masculine man with a conscious, open heart. His advice to women is also to play more and exercise their feminine.

Step 5: Thank Your Lucky Stars. Gratitude is present in Casey's every word. The courage to share his story is also evidence of his gratitude. Without the journey, he would not have found his love.

All women and men can benefit from Casey's consciousness and courage. It starts with a decision to clean up your life, look in the mirror and be honest about what may be holding you back. It then takes self-love and respect to dive into the shadow parts of yourself and trust that you are whole and perfect just the way you are. When Casey felt *good enough*, something we all struggle with in our lives, he could then open up the space to attract exactly what he pictured in his mind.

Chapter 14

Your 4-Week Plan

"Your persistence is your belief in yourself." **Brian Tracy**

Grab a notebook or piece of paper and write down the things you are willing to do for each step, each week. Post the piece of paper somewhere you can see it as a reminder to take action. Plan out your action steps for the first week to start with a loose plan of what you would like to accomplish for each week thereafter. Once you get started, you may change your mind or find an unexpected momentum. Be willing to be flexible—just stay in action. Week 1 is about getting started, and you should progress at your own pace through week 2, 3, and 4.

Week 1

Step 1: Clean the Slate
Start by choosing one area of your life to clean up: body, physical environment, or emotions. If you are someone who resists this kind of change, pick something easy that you are willing to do, like clean off your desk. Prepare the bedroom for someone else to join and support you. Make space in your closet. Create space with an empty bedside table on the other side of the bed for your future mate. Clean up the room and create a romantic atmosphere. If you are ready for some major changes, do a detox. The consuming nature of a detox will motivate you to do smaller tasks while cleansing your body; you can get a lot accomplished in nine or ten days.

Step 2: Sexual Fitness

Change one thing about your workout routine. Adding isometrics to your upper and lower body can get you started quickly on gaining extra stamina. Not working out at all? Sign up for a Pilates class or join a gym that offers classes. Get your body moving somehow and start now!

Step 3: A Food Love Affair

The fastest way to reconnect with your food is to cook it and prepare it yourself. Schedule one meal a day that you make with your hands. Take the time to clean, chop, and cook. Leave enough time to sit down at a table and eat the food without any distractions: no TV or computer. Spend some quality, loving time with your food.

Step 4: Wear Sexy Underwear

Look through the sexy clothes, underwear, and lingerie that you already have right now. Choose something to wear around the house before bedtime and even sleep in it. As you are exploring your underwear drawer, throw out anything old, ripped, stained, or anything that does not fit. If that leaves you with only a few things, then it is time to go shopping! Start adorning yourself somehow every day.

Step 5: Thank Your Lucky Stars

Take out a journal or piece of paper, write in big letters at the top: GRATITUDE LIST. Stick it next to your bed or even on your bed to remind you to start this today. You can keep using the same piece of paper or get a proper journal to keep on the bedside table every night.

Week 2

Step 1: Clean the Slate

Clean out your refrigerator and pantry. Take out everything that you can live without. Throw out the things that are not serving you or give them away. Make a trip to the grocery store and load up on vegetables. Plan to eat at least 2 to 3 servings of vegetables every day.

Step 2: Sexual Fitness
Add at least one day of steady state training cardio to your week and 20 to 30 minutes of abs. Start researching dance classes in your area that would interest you.

Step 3: A Food Love Affair
Plant an herb. No matter where you live, caring for a small potted herb is possible for all of us. When you are at the grocery store buying your vegetables, smell test the herbs and find one you really love. Basil is an aphrodisiac and can be used in many dishes. Try it if you are looking for something new and exciting.

Step 4: Wear Sexy Underwear
Buy yourself your favorite flower. If you do not have a favorite, buy at least one dozen roses. Spend a few minutes cutting them and arranging them in a vase. Be sure to place them either in your bedroom or on your dining room table. The energy of the flowers should be like the energy of another person saying *good morning* or *hello, beautiful* to you every day.

Step 5: Thank Your Lucky Stars
Make a list of all your favorite people in your life and write down why they are important to you. Be very detailed and do not leave anything out. Keep adding to the list people you remember as you do this each week.

Week 3

Step 1: Clean the Slate
If you haven't already done so, schedule at least a five-day detox. Doing it during the workweek might provide enough distractions for you to focus on other things while you are making these big shifts in your diet during this time. Start to make a list or notice the people you spend time with that suck your energy and change your mood. Notice how they interact with other people, as well. Choose to spend time with people you feel good around and those that see the world through more positive eyes.

Step 2: Sexual Fitness

Last week, you were to research a dance class nearby that interested you. This week, go to that class! Call ahead and ask about the dress code so you can be prepared. Bring more than one kind of shoes, as each dance floor and kinds of dance have different footwear needs. If you are not ready for this, take a new group fitness class at a gym or tune into a dance fitness class on your TV at home.

Step 3: A Food Love Affair

Play a game with your food: eat from the color of the rainbow everyday in fruits and vegetables. Find different ways of preparing them and eating them. Pack them in a bag for lunch and to have as a snack. Before you eat it, hold it in your hands, take a breath, and give thanks for all involved to bring this vegetable to you. When you can take five minutes before inhaling your food to be present with it, your hunger will actually decrease and your satisfaction will increase. It's amazing how much I love eating veggies with people who treat each piece of produce like gold.

Step 4: Wear Sexy Underwear

Make a date with a friend to do something you would do with a partner, minus the intimacy. I'd prefer you focus on a male friend to satisfy your feminine need for masculine polarity. If you are lacking in male companionship, gather some of the girls and head out to a sporting event. Soak up the masculine energy by just being around it, but remember not to match it. Attraction is created by polarity: opposites attract. Recalibrate your energy and activate the woman inside!

Step 5: Thank Your Lucky Stars

From your list of favorite people, write one of them a note. Share with them why they are important to you and send it to them. A note is better than a phone call because they can read it over and over as often as they want. It is a true gift to give someone when you let him or her know you appreciate them. You will find you feel appreciated more by those around you when you start the cycle of appreciation energy.

Week 4

Step 1: Clean the Slate

Be willing to let go of things in your life, including people that are not serving you any longer. Take a good look around your home, office, car, and work for what just doesn't *fit* with who you want to become. Since this is often very hard to do, make a list and start with the easiest first. Journal about it and have closure. In Feng Shui, there are three questions to ask before tossing something away that will determine if it stays or if it goes. These questions are: Do you love it? Do you use it? Do you need it? If you answer yes to any one of them, keep it. As long as you become aware of what needs to go, you can allow the time and space for clues to let you know when you are ready to let it go.

Step 2: Sexual Fitness

Self-pleasure. If this is something that makes you uncomfortable, start with simple actions, like taking a bubble bath. Set the scene in your tub with rose petals or lavender in the water, candles lit along the side, and maybe a glass of tea or wine to enjoy while you soak. Plan a spa day with some girlfriends or alone. I love both. When I want to retreat from the world completely, I take a book and go to the spa for several hours alone. Since I speak to people all day, I find it refreshing to be somewhere where silence is expected. Spa days with my girlfriends are also a treat for my mind, body, and soul. Go to a naked spa; if you are wearing clothes, stay home and save your money until you are ready.

Step 3: A Food Love Affair

Take a cooking class. Whole Foods Market and Williams Sonoma stores have locations that offer cooking classes where you prepare and cook the food, as well as free demos where the crowd gets to watch, learn, and sample. My husband and I did a few on a Sunday morning at Williams Sonoma and were introduced to a whole new world of salt and spices. I found truffle salt, which is an aphrodisiac to me and has heightened my sense of cooking and spices ever since. Go alone or take a friend. It's a fine time to learn about food.

Step 4: Wear Sexy Underwear

Take a trip to Victoria's Secret and get yourself at least one new set of underwear and a sexy *nightie*. The first step is having *it*; the next step is wearing it. Play with the experience of trying all the different choices. If you are unwilling to make the time right now to go to the store, grab or order a Victoria's Secret catalogue. You can flip through it while you are in the bathroom. Make a plan to spice up your inner wardrobe.

Step 5: Thank Your Lucky Stars

The exercise this week is the most important, and I think you are ready. Take 20 minutes and stand in front of the mirror. Resist any urge to criticize yourself. Aloud, I want you to tell yourself what you appreciate about you in every aspect: your body, mind, heart, spirit, and soul. I want you to say *thank you* to every part of you that makes you who you are. Take this very seriously, but be playful with an open heart. Use your most open, loving heart when speaking to yourself, as if you were talking to a small child. When you are done, write yourself a love letter including all the things that came up for you in this exercise. Seal it and put it in special place.

In every section, there are several suggestions for each step. This four-week plan is designed to easily move you through each step. Depending upon your level of readiness, feel free to adjust it. My goal is to support your process, not create resistance to it. Whatever you choose will be the right choice. Revisit this book and these steps at least once a quarter to make sure you are moving forward on your journey. I have listed a number of resources for further exploration. Reach out for support when you need it. It's a sign of self-respect and love to ask for help. Contact me at invisiblefitness.com if you need some assistance with creating your perfect 4 week plan.

Resources

Books

For Your Body

Knack Absolute Abs: Routines for a Fit and Firm Core by JJ Flizanes

The 150 Healthiest Foods on Earth by Dr. Jonny Bowden

Inter Courses: an aphrodisiac cookbook by Martha Hopkins

The Most Decadent Diet Ever by Devin Alexander

The 5 Minute Diet by Ajay Rochester

For Your Relationships

If Love is Game, These are the Rules by Dr. Cherie Carter-Scott

If Life is a Game, These are the Rules by Dr. Cherie Carter-Scott

Keys to the Kingdom by Alison Armstrong

Women, Food and God by Geneen Roth

Dear Lover by David Deida

Way of the Superior Man by David Deida

Building Your Field of Dreams by Mary Manin Morrissey

Workshops

Fit 2 Love 2 Day Workshop: fit2love.info/workshop

Sex, Passion, and Enlightenment: warriorsage.com

Celebrating Men, Satisfying Women:	PAX, celebratingmen.com
Understanding Men:	PAX, celebratingmen.com
Warrior Camp:	peakpotentials.com

Products

Fit 2 Love Sexual Fitness Exercises:	fit2love.info/exercises
The 6 Week Beach Body Program:	6weekbeachbody.com/F2L
30 Day JUMP Start Program (*free*):	invisiblefitness.com
90 Day Health and Body Makeover:	invisiblefitness.com/90Day
Today: The Daily Journal:	thehotproject.com
9 Day Detox:	jjsdetox.com
Slimware:	skinnyplates.info

Websites

Mayo Clinic:	mayoclinic.org
JJ's Ab Book:	jjsabbook.com
Nourishing Wellness:	nourishingwellness.com
Coe-Dynamics Pilates:	coe-dynamics.com
Life & Relationship Coach:	carolchanel.com
Graphic Design:	gregalbers.com
Web Solutions:	everyanglemedia.com

More info about featured stories

Brian Albers: brian.albers@hotmail.com

Jody Lay: hansenengineering.com

Jennifer Torok: wingsandrootswellness.com

Mike Burrichter: cbre.com

Alexis Neely: alexisneely.com

Casey Capshaw: caseycapshaw.com

About the Author

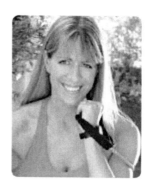

Credentials and accolades follow the name of JJ Flizanes wherever it appears, and for good reason. JJ, author of *Knack Absolute Abs: Routines for a Fit and Firm Core*, is *America's Guilt Free Trainer* and the creator of world-class fitness programs and routines, such as the Foundations Program for the New York Sports Club and Invisible Fitness®. What sets JJ apart from her Celebrity Fitness counterparts lies in her anatomically-centered routines, which protect overworked and aging joints from catastrophic failure and the integration of mind, body, and spirit.

Named Best Personal Trainer in Los Angeles for 2007 by *Elite Traveler Magazine*, JJ has been lauded by *Shape Magazine* as one of the top fitness trainers in 2003. Flizanes was also chosen by the fitness industry as IDEA Personal Trainer of the Year finalist for 2010. As a leader in innovative exercise, JJ has been certified by the National Academy of Sports Medicine (NASM) and also served as a Continuing Education Provider.

JJ launched her professional career in 1996 as the Foundations Director for the New York Sports Club, where she designed curriculum and in-house certification for new and previously uncertified fitness trainers. She has also been certified by the American Council on Exercise (ACE), International Sports Science Association (ISSA), and the Resistance Training Specialist Program (RTS).

With a focus on biomechanics, JJ has lectured for The Learning Annex and as a featured speaker for New York Times Bestselling Author of *The Millionaire Mind*, T. Harv Ecker's *Peak Potentials* seminars, as well as corporate clients, including Pacific Gas and Electric, Hanson Engineering, and Jostens, Inc. She is the Wellness Expert for FKC International, the Health and Fitness Expert for the National Association of Entrepreneur Moms, and a Fitness Expert for Nourishing Wellness Medical Center.

A favorite of journalists and the media for her depth of knowledge and vibrant personality, JJ, a regular contributing expert for *Get Active Magazine*, has also been featured in many national magazines, including *Women's Health*, *Muscle and Fitness HERS*, *Elegant Bride*, *Fitness Magazine*, and *E Pregnancy Magazine*, to name a few. Her television appearances include LA's KTLA, FOX 11, CBS, and NBC.

In June of 2009, JJ introduced her most challenging and exciting program: *The 6 Week Beach Body Program*, in which candidates take on creating a new body and lifestyle for life. Invisible Fitness offers personal training, fitness coaching, corporate programs, workshops, and seminars. For program details, please contact the office at 1.800.571.5722 or at <u>invisiblefitness.com</u>.

LaVergne, TN USA
09 February 2011
215975LV00003B/75/P